Allergies
Answers at your fingertips

Dr Joanne Clough DM, FRCA, MRCP, FRCPCH

CLASS PUBLISHING · LONDON

Printing history
First published 1997
Reprinted with amendments 1998
Second edition 2007

The information presented in this book is accurate and current to the best of the author's knowledge. The author and publisher, however, make no guarantee as to, and assume no responsibility for, the correctness, sufficiency or completeness of such information or recommendation. The reader is advised to consult a doctor regarding all aspects of individual health care.

The author and the publisher welcome feedback from the users of this book. Please contact the publisher.

Class Publishing (London) Ltd, Barb House, Barb Mews, London W6 7PA
Telephone: 020 7371 2119 / Fax: 020 7371 2878
Email: post@class.co.uk
Visit our website: www.class.co.uk

A CIP record for this book is available from the British Library.

ISBN 13: 978 1 85959 147 5
ISBN 10: 1 85959 147 7

10 9 8 7 6 5 4 3 2 1

Edited by Gillian Clarke
Illustrations by David Woodroffe
Cartoons by Jane Taylor
Index by Vicki Robinson

Designed and typeset by Martin Bristow

Printed and bound in Finland by WS Bookwell, Juva

Comments on *Allergies: answers at your fingertips* from readers

'I found the text extremely enjoyable and informative. I am sure that her readers will find Dr Clough's style both easily readable and accessible – I wish I could write this succinctly!'

SUE OLLIER
Scientific Director, British Allergy Foundation
(now Allergy UK)

'. . . a clear, informative and authoritative book which provides a useful source of information for all those with asthma, hay fever, eczema, anaphylaxis and other allergies.'

DR MARTYN PARTRIDGE
Chief Medical Adviser, National Asthma Campaign

'The small (even silly) questions you have answered are often the ones that can cause the most stress and are impossible to get answered by the medical profession.'

MRS CALLA FLEISCHER
London

'An invaluable reference source.'

NIKKI LANCASTER
Children's Outpatient Department,
Southampton General Hospital

'This really is a very excellent book, and has a very excellent index.'
DR A W FRANKLAND DM, FRCP

'I am sure it will be of great help to many patients.'
PROFESSOR JONATHAN BROSTOFF
Professor of Allergy and Environmental Health,
The Middlesex Hospital

'I think that it is excellent. It is very clearly written and provides extremely useful information which I am sure will benefit allergy sufferers. I shall recommend it to all my patients.'

'The book will, I am sure, be of as much value to health professionals as to the patients under their care.'

Reviews of *Allergies: answers at your fingertips*

'Gives sensible, practical advice on all the questions you might have about allergies – what they are, how they develop and, most importantly, how to deal with them.'

'A useful section on anaphylaxis'

'Essential reading for allergy sufferers'

'. . . gives no-nonsense, medically accurate answers to hundreds of questions asked by people with allergies.'

'. . . answers questions from people affected by allergies – giving factual info on eczema, dermatitis, hay fever, and both mild and strong food allergies.'

Contents

About the author

Dr Joanne Clough DM, FRCA, MRCP, FRCPCH is a paediatric physician specialising in asthma and allergic diseases. She was formerly a Senior Lecturer at the University of Southampton and a Consultant at Southampton General Hospital. She is a Fellow of the Royal College of Paediatrics & Child Health, a Member of the Royal College of Physicians and a member of the British Society for Allergy and Clinical Immunology. She now works as a Medical Adviser, and was closely involved in *Food Allergies* by Tanya Wright and in the UK editions of *Managing Your Arthritis* and *Managing Arthritis Pain* from the US Arthritis Foundation, all published by Class.

Acknowledgements

I am grateful to everyone who has helped in the production of this book, but in particular thank the following:

Jane Taylor, for drawing such delightful cartoons;

Education for Health, for providing the line illustrations of devices that appear in Chapter 2;

members of Allergy UK, for passing on to me questions and queries on allergy problems;

my editor, Gillian Clarke, for her impeccable editing and unflagging enthusiasm;

and finally my patients and friends who have allergy disorders, for providing me with many of the questions and most of the answers.

Foreword

by **Professor Stephen T. Holgate** MD, DSc, FRCP
MRC Clinical Professor of Immunopharmacology,
University of Southampton

The word allergy is often used broadly to describe some type of 'sensitivity' to environmental factors, but this is too loose a description. The term was first used in 1906 by Pirquet, who used it to describe an immunological reaction against substances in our environment. Nowadays the term 'allergy' is used specifically to indicate harmful reactions to substances in our everyday environment which produce their effect through mechanisms involving the immune response, leading to various types of acute or chronic inflammation and the symptoms that ensue. This definition of allergy separates it, quite clearly, from the many other forms of intolerance that occur to environmental substances, such as reactions to food causing migraine and irritable bowel syndrome.

One of the common features of allergic disorders is that they tend to cluster in families and, in any one person, may manifest at a number of organ sites. For example, it is quite common for someone to have asthma, food allergy, hay fever and eczema together. Thus allergy tends not to affect a single organ but multiple organs, producing a range of symptoms. It is because of this that allergy fits uncomfortably into the more traditional practice of medicine in the UK, in which disease specialists treat conditions centred in particular systems or organs.

This book is a refreshing distillation of the medical literature, written in a question and answer format and designed to help steer patients accurately through the allergy maze. Dr Clough is a child health specialist who has a special interest in allergic disease, and she is therefore particularly well qualified to translate medical knowledge into a form that is easily understandable by the general public. The rising trends that appear to be occurring in disorders such as asthma and hay fever are almost entirely related to the increasing trends in allergy probably produced by changes in our environment. The importance of environment in helping allergic disorder cannot be underestimated. This book presents a balanced view of how medical intervention coupled with environmental control can lead to improvement in the manifestations of many allergic disorders.

The continued high prevalence of asthma and allergy remains a concern, as does the rising trends in developing countries. The fragmented and often rudimentary knowledge of allergy in its diagnosis and management is problematic in a health service such as ours, which tends to treat disease on an organ basis. The very practical and sensible approach that Dr Clough has taken in this book, now in its second edition, will, I am sure, be helpful both to those who experience allergic reactions themselves and to their families. Whilst the book is not intended as a substitute for consultation with general practitioners or a hospital-based specialist, it certainly does produce excellent first-hand guidance as to what those affected can do when confronted by the myriad symptoms linked to allergic disorders and what they can do to prevent or control symptoms.

Stephen T. Holgate

Introduction

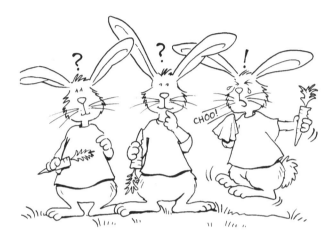

Allergy is extremely common, with one in three of the UK population now suffering from a medical condition caused by or associated with allergy – a total of 18 million people. As many as half of all sufferers are children. In any one year, 12 million people in the UK will seek medical help for their allergies, and half of these have problems that are severe enough to warrant the care of a specialist in allergy. Since the 1990s, hospital admissions for allergy have increased three-fold. However, allergy services in the UK are inadequate, and expert advice and treatment is very difficult to access, as there are only eight allergy clinics run by specialists in allergy in the UK. In 2006 the Department of Health published *A review of services for allergy*, which highlighted this problem and made a number of recommendations. Until these recommendations come into effect, it is more important than ever that individuals affected by allergy do their best to become well informed about their condition and its treatment. The aim of this book is to help you do this.

Despite these problems being so common, misunderstandings about allergy are frequent and misinformation is rife. The enormous number of different ways in which allergic disorders can present themselves may be partly responsible for this confusion: an allergy may occur as an isolated problem such as penicillin allergy; it may be a part of one of the common allergic disorders of the Western world such as asthma, hay fever and eczema; or it may be associated with a less common problem such as a workplace allergy, for example latex allergy. Some sufferers may be allergic to only one substance, others to a wide variety. The problems caused by allergy may be trivial (such as nettle rash) or they may be life-threatening (such as anaphylaxis). Despite these differences, it is the same underlying biological mechanism that is responsible for each of these many different conditions.

Another thing that many people with allergic disease have in common is that they suffer from chronic low-level symptoms that, although subtle, may have a considerable impact on their everyday lives. Poor-quality sleep and not enough of it; a blocked or itchy nose; bad breath; a scratchy throat; itchy and unsightly skin; poor appetite; decreased attention span; niggling abdominal symptoms – allergy sufferers often develop low expectations and believe that these symptoms, which may lead to increased time off work or school, are inevitable. But they are not!

Although we don't know everything about allergy, in the 21st century we are lucky that we do have a mine of information and some excellent new medications that anyone with an allergy-related problem will find invaluable in managing their disorder. The more you know about your condition, the more effectively you and your doctor will be able to tackle your allergy problems. Family and friends will also benefit from reading this book, as they may then feel more able to offer support and to co-operate with any necessary changes in your lifestyle.

Accurate diagnosis of what is and is not allergy is important: you may realise from reading this book that your problem is not due to allergy, in which case you will then be free to discover the real cause and seek appropriate treatment.

I hope that this book will help you to understand how and why allergies happen, what the common triggers are and how to manage your symptoms effectively, as well as dispelling some of the many myths about allergy that abound. If you are well informed and well prepared, you will feel more in control, your allergies will become more manageable and you will regain the ability to enjoy life to the full.

How to use this book

Because individual people have very different allergy problems, this book has been designed so that you do not have to read it from cover to cover unless you wish to do so. Instead, it can be used selectively to meet your own particular situation. It has a detailed list of contents and a comprehensive index so that you can quickly identify the parts that are relevant to you. Cross-references in the text will lead you to more detailed information when this might be useful, and essential information is repeated whenever it seems necessary.

Please remember that a book like this cannot provide exact and full answers to your individual health problems. What it can do, though, is provide you with enough information to help you seek out the answers from your doctors and other health professionals.

Not everyone will agree with all the answers I have given, but future editions of this book can be improved only if you let me know where you disagree or have found the advice to be unhelpful, or if you have any questions that you think I have not covered. Please write to me c/o Class Publishing, Barb House, Barb Mews, London W6 7PA, UK.

1 | What is allergy?

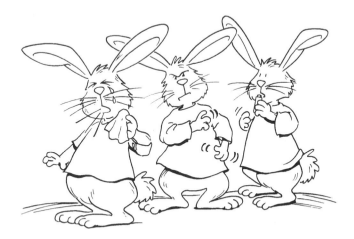

Allergy is becoming more common – the number of people affected in the UK has increased three-fold over the past 20 years. The reason for this is not entirely clear, but I explore some of the possibilities in this chapter. First of all, I want to explain what happens in the body when an allergy occurs, what the symptoms are, and how to decide whether or not an allergy is the cause of your own particular problem. In other sections of this chapter, I discuss some of the common substances that can set off the train of events leading to allergy, and answer the questions that are frequently asked about how allergy is inherited.

ALLERGY EXPLAINED

Allergy is a term that seems to be used to describe almost any kind of illness these days. What exactly is allergy?

If you have an allergy, your immune system reacts abnormally or inappropriately to a substance that should be harmless. Our immune system is a complex defence network that has developed to protect us from a number of different threats, including cancer cells and outside 'attackers' such as viruses and bacteria, many of which would otherwise be fatal. The immune system is made up of a considerable number of different cell types and chemical 'messengers', which work together in a co-ordinated way to identify and destroy these invaders.

In some individuals, the immune system over-reacts, and responds to a harmless substance as if it is a threat. The resulting chain of events is what we know of as an allergic reaction.

The term 'allergy' is often used rather loosely to describe any unpleasant reaction of the body to a food or a drug, but many of these reactions (e.g. nausea after taking certain antibiotics, or diarrhoea in toddlers when they eat certain foods) are due to a predictable effect and are not allergic in origin.

True allergic reactions always involve the production of IgE, the allergy antibody. They tend to occur in people who are prone to allergic disorders (e.g. asthma and hay fever), a tendency which is described as atopy.

What exactly is atopy?

Atopy is not an illness. It is an inherited characteristic which makes a person more likely to develop an allergic disorder. You may not know yet that you are atopic, as not everyone who is atopic actually has one of the allergic disorders – which include asthma, eczema and hay fever – but all atopic people have inherited the tendency or predisposition to develop them, and might do so in the future.

The reason why atopic people have a tendency to develop allergic disorders is that they have the ability to produce the allergy antibody (called immunoglobulin E, or IgE; discussed in more detail in the answer to the next question) when they come into contact with common substances that would not normally be harmful. The word atopy is a good way of describing this inappropriate reaction, as it is derived from the Greek word *atopos*, which means 'out of place'.

The common allergic diseases are asthma, hay fever, eczema and food allergy. There are other conditions, not dependent on IgE, in which other abnormal immune responses cause disease; for example, certain forms of contact dermatitis and coeliac disease.

Atopy is a characteristic that tends to run in families, and a number of scientists are currently trying to identify the genes on our chromosomes that cause it (genes determine the characteristics we inherit from our parents, and chromosomes are the structures in our body cells that carry the genes). Identifying the genes would make it easier to carry out research into why allergies happen, how they are inherited and what we can do to prevent them. In the meantime, your doctor makes the diagnosis of atopy mainly by paying attention to the symptoms you describe, perhaps with the help of some of the tests described in Appendix 1.

How do you become allergic to something?

To explain this, I need to start by describing how the immune system works. The immune system is the network within the body that protects us from outside 'attackers', which include viruses, bacteria and parasites. This system is usually very efficient at telling the difference between these harmful micro-organisms and other harmless substances that do not pose a threat to your body.

When your immune system defends your body against a potentially harmful attacker for the first time, it not only fights the infection but also develops a memory of the micro-organism, so that it can be recognised if it attacks you again. This memory, which is life-long, is in the form of many small structures called antibodies. Each set of antibodies is unique, having been tailor-made to fit that attacker, and you develop a different set of antibodies for each new attacker.

There are five different types or classes of antibody. Each type, termed an immunoglobulin, has a different function:

- Immunoglobulin A (abbreviation IgA) is found in secretions such as tears and saliva, and defends us against micro-organisms that might invade our respiratory and digestive systems.

- Immunoglobulin M (IgM) is a temporary type of antibody

formed when a new attacker invades our body, which protects us until IgG can be made.

- Immunoglobulin G (IgG) is the antibody that takes over from IgM to form a lasting (usually life-long) memory of the attacker.

- Immunoglobulin D (IgD) is a mystery – we know it is there but we do not know what it does.

- Immunoglobulin E (IgE) is the allergy antibody. People who do not have allergies normally have only tiny amounts of IgE but can produce more when needed – for example, as a response to a parasitic infection. People with allergies readily produce large amounts of IgE.

The first time you meet a harmful organism, it takes the immune system a few days to mount a response. However, if your immune system is working effectively, it will then be constantly at the ready to recognise and eliminate the same attacker if it meets it again. If this happens, the tailor-made IgG antibodies, which have already been made, attach immediately to the attacker, allowing the many other components of the immune system, led by the white blood cells, to go into action. Some of these cells produce chemical messengers which alert other cells in the immune system that an 'attack' is happening and encourage them to gather. Another group of cells produces chemicals (including histamine) that increase the 'leakiness' of the blood vessels to allow white blood cells to move out of the blood vessels and into the tissues where they can fight the 'attackers'. The whole process is very efficient, which is why we suffer only once from each childhood infection such as chickenpox.

If you are atopic, your immune system works perfectly well against these infectious organisms. However, it also has a tendency to over-react to substances that should be harmless, and to treat them as if they were attackers. These substances, known as allergens, can come into contact with the body's immune system by various routes, including being inhaled, swallowed or injected (as in a wasp sting), or coming into contact with the skin or eye. They are mistakenly seen by your immune system as being dangerous, and antibodies of the type known as immunoglobulin E (IgE) are made against them.

Once your body has met and become sensitised to an allergen, large amounts of IgE are quickly made when it meets even tiny amounts of the same allergen again. The IgE allows the allergen to attach itself to a number of different cells of the immune system. This IgE then sets off a complex series of events, which we know as an allergic reaction. This process involves many other components of the immune system, particularly the white blood cells, all of which are co-ordinated by the body's chemical messengers. The end result of this complex chain of events is that large quantities of chemicals, including histamine, are produced in the tissues, which cause swelling, redness, soreness and itching. Other cells are encouraged to produce more IgE antibodies that will, in their turn, be able to continue the inflammatory process.

An allergy cannot happen the first time you come into contact with an allergen – you first have to become sensitised to it. Sensitisation does not produce any symptoms, and you will not be aware that it has happened. You may tolerate a substance quite happily for a long time and then, for no apparent reason, develop an allergic reaction to it. Once this has happened, an allergic response will take place each time your body meets that allergen, even in minute amounts. Your reaction will not necessarily be identical on each occasion: there are many factors that may alter its severity, and the allergy may grow weaker – or indeed stronger – with time. You can see that allergies are not very predictable!

I know that allergies are often treated with antihistamine medicines, but what is histamine?

Histamine is just one (but probably the best known) of the chemicals produced by your body in the course of an allergic reaction, and it causes the symptoms of itching, swelling, redness and mucus production. It is produced by your body as the end result of a large number of messages that are passed in chemical form from one cell to another, a process that begins when your body comes into contact with an allergen.

As you say, one of the treatments for allergies is to give drugs that block the action of histamine, called antihistamines. Whilst these drugs can be extremely useful, they only suppress the effects of histamine after it has been produced. Treatments that interrupt the allergy process at an earlier stage, before the chemicals that cause inflammation are produced, are usually more effective. Such treatments include the steroid preparations used in asthma and eczema.

What is an allergen? How many different allergens are there?

An allergen is any substance that acts as a trigger for allergy, provoking an allergic reaction in someone who is atopic (allergic reactions and atopy are discussed in more detail in the section called 'Allergy explained' at the beginning of this chapter).

The most common allergens are house dust mites, pollen from trees and grasses, foods such as peanut and egg proteins, moulds and spores, and animal allergens such as dog dander (the scales from their hair or fur, something like dandruff in humans), and cat dander (a combination of saliva, which cats use for grooming, and their skin scales). What these all have in common is that they contain protein: for example, the house dust mite allergen is a protein found in the mite faeces; pollen is a protein; and there is a protein found in cat saliva. In foods, it is only the protein fragments that can cause allergies – if peanut oil is 100% pure oil (containing only the oil and no protein fragments) it will not cause peanut allergy. Although we tend to think of protein as part of the food we eat, a protein is in fact an organic compound containing hydrogen, oxygen and nitrogen and which forms an important part of all living organisms. There are many, many different proteins, and their importance to life is shown in the name: the word 'protein' comes from the Greek word *proteios*, which means 'primary'.

There are some non-protein allergens, including penicillin and some other drugs. In order to cause an allergy, these have to be bound to a protein once they are in the body.

It is impossible to say how many different allergens exist: as well as the more common ones, rarer allergies can be to substances as wide ranging as castor oil plants and ladybird bites.

My doctor has told me that my bowel problems are caused by a food intolerance, but I'm sure it's all due to an allergy. Sometimes even the thought of certain foods makes me feel sick. My husband thinks I've just got a rather sensitive stomach. Are we all just using different words to describe the same thing, or is there really a difference between allergy, intolerance and sensitivity? And does it matter?

Although the term 'allergy' is commonly used to describe any unpleasant reaction to a drug, food, insect sting or chemical, it is more correct to reserve it for the description of true allergic reactions, and to use the terms aversion, intolerance and sensitivity as follows.

- *Aversion* to food happens in people who have had an unpleasant experience with a particular food, such as being very sick after eating a bad oyster. They believe that the same thing will happen each time they eat that food, and may feel unwell even when they only see or think of that food. They therefore avoid eating the food, although in reality they will come to no harm if they do (unless they are unlucky enough to be served another bad oyster!).

- An *intolerance* is said to occur when you develop unpleasant symptoms after eating a substance that your body cannot handle adequately. For example, some people have unpleasant symptoms after drinking milk or eating products made from milk. They cannot digest milk and milk products properly because their digestive systems do not produce enough of a particular enzyme called lactase, which is needed to break down and digest the sugar in the milk (called lactose). The symptoms include crampy abdominal pain, bloating and diarrhoea, all of which are due to the presence of undigested milk sugar in the bowel. These symptoms are not allergic in nature, and will not occur if only tiny quantities of milk are drunk (unlike an allergy). This form of food intolerance is called lactose intolerance, and the answer to it is to avoid all but very small quantities of milk and milk products in the diet.

- A *sensitivity* to a substance is a reaction that is an exaggeration of a normal side effect of that substance. For example, consider salbutamol (Ventolin and Aerolin) which is used in reliever inhalers for asthma. If it is given in a high enough dose, most people will develop shakiness and feel 'revved up'. Some individuals, particularly children, develop these side effects on quite small doses, and can be said to be unusually *sensitive* to salbutamol, but they are not allergic to it.

- A *true allergy* is a reaction produced when your body meets a normally harmless substance that it remembers from a previous exposure, and the reaction involves the production of IgE antibodies (these were discussed in an earlier answer in this section). Once an allergy has developed, even a tiny amount of the allergen can lead to a reaction.

The difference between intolerance, sensitivity and allergy can matter, because if your problem is not correctly diagnosed you may not get the most appropriate and effective treatment for it – for example, antihistamine medications will not help if your problem is actually lactose intolerance. However, if you find that the only suitable treatment for your symptoms is to avoid the substance that is affecting you, it probably doesn't matter which term you use. In your particular case, it sounds as if you know that there are particular foods that upset you, and you may want to eliminate them from your diet.

If you decide to eliminate whole food groups, such as dairy foods, do please get the help of a registered dietitian, who will make sure you are not going to suffer from a nutritional deficiency.

You will find more information about food allergies in Chapter 5, and about allergen avoidance in Chapter 9.

I have hay fever that affects my nose, my eyes and my chest. I have a friend who has an allergy that affects her skin. Are there any other parts of the body that can be affected by allergies?

Allergic reactions can occur as a generalised reaction involving the skin (urticaria, angioedema) or the whole body (anaphylaxis), or they may be confined to specific parts of the body such as the eyes (allergic conjunctivitis, hay fever), the nose (perennial allergic rhinitis, hay fever), the lungs (asthma), the skin (eczema, contact dermatitis) or the bowel (food allergies). The symptoms of the allergic reaction will vary depending upon which part of the body is affected, but the underlying mechanism of what is happening in the immune system is the same for all of them.

The allergies mentioned here are discussed in other chapters in this book.

I have heard of people suffering from something called total allergy syndrome. What is this, how common is it, and how is it treated?

A number of different terms – including 'total allergy syndrome' and 'multiple chemical sensitivity' – are used to describe a condition in which the sufferer appears to experience reactions to a wide range of substances. The symptoms include memory loss, fatigue, depression, nausea and breathing difficulties. Because the substances thought to be responsible include many chemicals, plastics and other synthetics, this is sometimes regarded as an allergy to modern living. Sufferers often obtain some relief from their symptoms by avoiding exposure to all fumes and chemicals, but this often means that they end up cutting themselves off from everyday life.

Most doctors are reluctant to accept that this condition is in fact due to allergy, and certainly the classic immune response with the production of IgE (discussed earlier in this chapter) is not involved.

However, this does not mean to say that the symptoms are not real, just that they are not caused by allergy.

The Committee on Toxicity of Chemicals in Food, Consumer Products and the Environment (COT) is an independent scientific committee that provides advice to the Food Standards Agency, the Department of Health and other Government Departments and Agencies on matters concerning the toxicity of chemicals. In a recent report, it noted that there were 'no consistent patterns of symptoms or exposure data to define the condition of multiple chemical sensitivity', and concluded that, on the basis of knowledge current at the time, there was 'insufficient evidence to make comments on potential mechanisms or to recommend further research in this area'.

Clearly, learning more about multiple chemical sensitivity is not going to be easy: we are hampered by the absence of a clear definition of the problem, as there is no consistent pattern of symptoms. However, work on this debilitating condition continues in many countries.

If my allergies are not treated, will they become worse?

This is a difficult question to answer, as allergies can vary in their severity over relatively short periods of time, and many allergies become less severe as you grow older.

In some people, their allergy may increase in severity as time goes on, with repeated exposure to the allergen causing more marked symptoms each time. If you are one of these people, it is particularly important for you to avoid the allergen as much as you can, and to take any medications given to you exactly as prescribed by your doctor.

Chronic allergic inflammation can lead to thickening and scarring in the tissues affected, particularly in the lungs. This may produce more pronounced symptoms with loss of healthy lung tissue. If a safe and well-tolerated treatment is available for your allergy, it is better to treat it so that the inflammation is controlled and any scarring or other long-term consequences are kept to a minimum.

I am allergic to grass pollen. Will I always have this allergy?

Unfortunately the tendency to develop allergy (called atopy, and explained earlier in this chapter) is written as a permanent message on your chromosomes (the genetic material that you inherit from your parents) and will never go away. However, the likelihood of developing new allergies decreases with age, and often existing allergies become less troublesome as you grow older – elderly people seem to suffer fewer allergic problems. I don't know how old you are, but the good news is that, as you get older, your allergy is likely to become less of a problem.

As you know what is responsible for your allergy, you may be able to control your symptoms by minimising your contact with grass pollen (ways of doing this are discussed in the section 'Pollens' in Chapter 9). Alternatively, your symptoms might be reduced to relatively trouble-free levels by a careful choice from the wide range of treatments available, which you should discuss with your doctor. So, although you will probably always have the tendency to allergy, you need not always suffer the symptoms.

Can allergies be cured?

Most treatments for allergy aim to suppress the symptoms, but cannot cure the underlying disease. There is one treatment, called 'desensitisation' or 'allergen immunotherapy', which attempts to eliminate an allergy by making the body more tolerant of the allergen. To begin with, it is given (usually by injection) once, or perhaps twice, a week, starting with very low concentrations in minute doses. The concentration of the solution and the amounts given are increased slowly over a period of three to six months, until the highest planned dosage is reached. That dose is then repeated once a month to maintain the benefit, and this may have to continue for several years.

This is not a procedure to be undertaken lightly, as there are serious risks associated with it. In the near future, though, immunotherapy might become significantly safer. Using genetic modification techniques, allergens can be modified so that they are much less potent as an allergen yet are still recognised by the immune system when used for desensitisation. This work is still in the experimental stage.

Is it possible to vaccinate against allergy in the same way that is done for other diseases?

Any vaccine against allergy would have to work in the opposite way to conventional vaccines. Vaccines against infectious diseases such as measles work by switching the immune system on and stimulating it to produce protective antibodies. To be able to vaccinate against allergy, we would need to switch *off* the immune system, to prevent it from producing IgE against allergens.

One approach would be to vaccinate people who have already developed an allergy. One research team has genetically engineered the pollen of birch trees so that, in the bodies of allergy sufferers, it produces antibodies that greatly reduce the immune response. If this could be given to people with birch allergy, it might reduce the intensity of their allergic reaction to normal (unmodified) birch pollen. However, this type of treatment is still in the very early stages of development.

An even better technique would be to develop a vaccine against allergy that might be used to protect children from developing allergies. Research in this area is going on at the moment. If this is successful, the vaccine (made from a micro-organism related to the tuberculosis organism) could be given to babies before they had the chance to become allergic to anything. Unfortunately, such a vaccine is still a long way from commercial production and, as yet, we have no proof that it will be effective.

What is immunotherapy?

Immunotherapy (desensitisation) is a treatment that aims to reduce or even eliminate symptoms of specific allergies by making the body more tolerant of the allergen responsible. This is done by giving repeated injections of increasing amounts of the allergen, starting with minute doses. It is only effective against certain types of allergic disease such as hay fever, other seasonal allergies, and anaphylaxis caused by insect stings such as wasp and bee stings. It cannot be used against food and drug allergies, although it is sometimes used to provide temporary protection in rare cases of drug allergy where the drug in question is the only possible form of treatment for a serious illness. It is never appropriate for non-seasonal asthma or perennial allergic rhinitis, or for allergies of the digestive system or skin.

Immunotherapy may take many months to achieve results, and may even need to be a life-long therapy. It therefore requires a major commitment. Treatment begins with the injection, into the deeper layers of the skin, of a very small quantity of the substance to which you are allergic. Each time the injection is repeated, the quantity of the allergen is increased (provided that the previous injection did not produce undue symptoms), until a maintenance level is reached. This is one that, without producing problems itself, controls the symptoms of the allergy being treated. Injections are given once or twice a week at first, reducing to once a month after a few months. This treatment must only be given in a hospital by an allergy specialist, and, on each occasion, the person receiving treatment must be closely observed for a minimum of two hours, as a severe reaction can occur. This happens in between 3% and 12% of patients, is more common in children and in women rather than men, and is more likely if the person is being treated for bee-sting allergy.

A new form of immunotherapy is now available that does away with the need for injections. It takes the form of a pill, which is dissolved under the tongue once a day for eight weeks before the pollen season starts. Tests have shown that it cuts symptoms by up to 40% in over 80% of people who used it, and it is much safer than conventional immunotherapy. At present it is available only for use in hay fever due to grass pollen allergy but, in the future, other forms of the treatment might be developed to manage different allergies.

I hate injections! Is there any type of immunotherapy that doesn't involve needles?

A new form of specific immunotherapy has recently been developed, with increasing evidence of success: sublingual immunotherapy, given by drops of allergen solution under the tongue. The initial regimen of increasing doses (see the previous answer) still has to be given in hospital by allergy specialists, but maintenance doses can be administered by the patient at home. It is not as effective as conventional immunotherapy but the side effects are less severe. Most of the research work has been done in Italy but there are also large trials underway in the USA. The treatment may soon become available in the UK.

My daughter has always had very severe eczema. My doctor now tells me that she has something called hyper-IgE syndrome and has prescribed a drug that my husband takes for his ulcers! Can you explain this to me?

Hyper-immunoglobulin E syndrome (usually abbreviated to hyper-IgE) is a rare condition in which enormous amounts of the immunoglobulin E antibody are produced. This leads to an exaggerated tendency towards allergic disorders, particularly eczema and asthma. We know that histamine, a chemical produced by the body, plays a major role in this problem. That is why the treatment consists of blocking the effects of histamine with antihistamine medicines.

It is not enough just to use the conventional antihistamine medications generally used in hay fever, as these block only some of the actions of histamine. There are two different cell receptors for histamine – H_1 and the H_2 receptors – and the anti-allergy antihistamines block only the H_1 receptors. Luckily, a second type of medication has been developed that blocks the other actions of histamine. These H_2 blockers are commonly used to treat stomach and duodenal (peptic) ulcers. Treatment for hyper-IgE consists of a combination of these two types of antihistamines: a conventional antihistamine such as ketotifen or cetirizine (both H_1 blockers) plus an ulcer drug such as cimetidine or ranitidine (both H_2 blockers). Do encourage your daughter to persevere with these medications, as it can take up to a year to see the full benefit, although she should begin to see some improvement within a few weeks.

SYMPTOMS

What are the symptoms of allergy, and how do they occur?

There is no such thing as a typical allergic reaction, as the symptoms can vary enormously between individuals, especially depending on the part of the body affected. The response to an allergen might even be different in the same person on two different occasions. To a certain extent, the symptoms you have will depend on which allergen is involved and which parts of your body are affected. A few examples are given here, but this list is not exhaustive.

- If grass pollen is the allergen, your eyes and nose will be affected. The pollen grains are relatively large and tend to settle on the surface of your eyes and the lining of your nose – which then become red and swollen, and produce an increased amount of secretions (i.e. you develop a runny nose and weepy eyes).

- A number of allergens – including those from house dust mites, cats and dogs – are very light, and so, instead of settling in your nose, they are inhaled down into your lungs, causing a narrowing of your airways. This leads to greater difficulty in moving air in and out of your airways, excess mucus or phlegm production (which blocks your airways even more) and increased irritability of your lungs causing coughing and wheezing.

- If your digestive system is affected by a food allergen, your bowel becomes inflamed and you will experience an increased volume of watery motions (diarrhoea) with spasm or colic of the bowel and sometimes vomiting.

Although these symptoms seem quite different from each other, they are all caused by the same process. Inflammation is your body's natural response when it feels it is under attack, and the process is designed to protect your body against the spread of an injury or infection. If you have an allergy, your body treats an allergen as an attacker, and sets up the inflammatory process. To start with, the allergen must gain access to your body, and this is usually through your nose, lungs or skin, or by mouth, into your bowel. Once there, the allergen is recognised by the specific IgE that was made the first time the allergen was encountered. The IgE allows the allergen to attach itself to a number of different cells of the immune system. Some of these cells produce chemical messengers that alert other cells in the immune system that an 'attack' is happening and encourage them to gather. Another group of cells produces chemicals (including histamine) that result in swelling, redness, soreness and itching. Without treatment, the inflammation may continue indefinitely, even after the allergen has been removed.

You will find more information about atopy and IgE antibodies in the section 'Allergy explained' at the beginning of this chapter.

How do I know if I am allergic to a particular allergen?

If you suspect that you might be allergic to something, it is likely that you have experienced a number of symptoms due to irritation or inflammation in one or more parts of your body. To decide whether an allergy is responsible, you should involve your doctor, who will need to consider:

- when your symptoms started;
- whether they occur at particular times of the day or year;
- how often they occur and how long they last;

- what makes your symptoms come on;

- which part of your body is affected;

- the type of symptoms you have and how severe they are;

- whether anyone else in your family has allergy-related problems;

- whether or not you have found anything that relieves your symptoms; and

- whether or not there is anything that makes them worse.

Sometimes the answers to these questions may not help much, because the symptoms and the trigger causing them aren't always clearly connected. The end result of an allergic reaction is inflammation of the affected part of the body, so the symptoms of allergy usually involve swelling, soreness, itchiness and increased secretions. But the symptoms of allergy can also be rather non-specific – for example, tiredness, irritability and moodiness. If your asthma is troublesome, you are likely to sleep less well and to feel tired and irritable as a consequence. However, generalised feelings of tiredness in the absence of specific allergic symptoms are unlikely to be due to allergy.

Food allergies can be particularly difficult to diagnose, because, once the allergen is absorbed from the bowel into the blood-stream, it can cause symptoms in several different parts of the body, including the lungs and the skin.

Also remember that one allergen may cause different symptoms in different people. One member of a family may sneeze and get watery eyes when they are with a cat, another may wheeze and cough.

Your doctor will then want to examine you. At this stage it might be clear whether your problem is due to an allergy. If not, you may be referred for further tests, which should give a definitive answer. (A number of different tests are used to look for evidence of particular allergies, and they are described in Appendix 1).

One indication that an allergy is responsible for your symptoms comes from seeing them improve when the allergen is removed from your environment or your diet. However, it is not always possible to avoid certain allergens, especially grass pollen and the house dust mite. If you are allergic to an allergen that cannot be avoided, your doctor will be able offer you one or more of the different medications currently available for the treatment of allergies.

My daughter is unwell whenever she drinks a lot of milk, which makes me think she may be allergic to it. However, my GP says it might not be an allergy but that she may just not be able to tolerate milk. He wants to perform some skin-prick tests, but as she is terrified of needles we are not very keen for her to have to go through that. Why can't our doctor simply tell what is wrong from her symptoms?

Most of the symptoms that our bodies produce as a way of telling us that something is wrong are not specific; that is, the same symptoms may be produced by a wide range of different problems or diseases. Because of this, your doctor cannot tell what is wrong with your daughter just from her symptoms. It sounds as if milk is certainly the cause, but whether her problem is an intolerance or an allergy will be difficult to tell without some form of testing. (The difference between intolerance and true allergy was discussed in the section 'Allergy explained' at the beginning of this chapter.)

The symptoms of milk intolerance (diarrhoea and abdominal discomfort) tend to occur only if relatively large amounts of milk are taken (small amounts are usually no problem) and the condition is often temporary. If a true allergy to milk is the problem (this usually occurs in younger children), the symptoms will occur even if only a tiny amount of milk is taken. However, the symptoms can be the same as those of milk intolerance.

Although my advice to you would be the same whichever the problem was – to avoid milk in your daughter's diet – I think that it is important to find out whether she has an *allergy*. If she does, you will need to be very strict with her diet and avoid milk completely, something that is not easy to do (just what is involved is discussed in the section 'Food allergens' in Chapter 9). If she has a milk *intolerance*, she will be able to take small quantities of milk, and will not be at risk of a dangerous reaction. Skin-prick testing (discussed further in Appendix 1) does not have to involve the use of needles. Small prongs called lancets are usually used, and these are only 1 mm long. Skin-prick testing does not hurt – I've had it done to see what it feels like – and can be done on your daughter's back if she prefers not to see what is happening. I would strongly advise that you allow your doctor to arrange these tests for your daughter so that you know how strict you need to be with her diet.

TRIGGERS

Why am I allergic to some things and not to others?

Being atopic does not mean that you will become allergic to any allergen in particular, just that you may, at some stage of your life, develop an allergy to something (atopy is discussed in more detail in the section 'Allergy explained' at the beginning of this chapter).

It seems that the way in which you first encounter an allergen is important in determining whether you will become allergic to it, as is the scale of your exposure to it. Factors that can make you more vulnerable to developing an allergy include being exposed to tobacco smoke or having a respiratory infection at the time. Because there are still many aspects of allergy that remain a mystery, we have no way of predicting whether you will develop any further allergies.

I have seen a number of advertisements for anti-house dust mite sprays. What is the house dust mite? Does it cause allergies?

The house dust mite is a species of small mite, too small to be seen with the naked eye, which lives on the scales of dead human skin that we are all constantly shedding. Its Latin name is *Dermato-phagoides pteronyssinus*, and it is the commonest type of mite living in house dust, although up to 12 different mite species can be found if the dust is analysed carefully. House dust mites are found in almost all homes in the UK, because they love the relatively warm and humid conditions found in British homes. We tend to insulate and draught-proof our homes in order to cut our heating bills, and the reduced level of ventilation that results produces ideal conditions for the mites to multiply. They especially like the insides of mattresses, pillows and soft furnishings, and also thrive inside children's cuddly toys.

It is not the mites themselves that cause allergies but their faecal particles (droppings). These particles are approximately the same size as small pollen grains, and can become air-borne for considerable periods of time, during which they may be inhaled. Increased exposure to the house dust mite may be responsible for at least some of the increase that we have seen over the past 20 years in the number of people suffering from asthma, eczema and perennial allergic rhinitis. We know that between 70% and 80% of people with asthma and rhinitis are allergic to the house dust mite, making it a major trigger factor of exacerbations as well.

Different ways of reducing the number of house dust mites in the home, including the sprays you mention, are discussed in Chapter 9.

What caused my asthma?

When we think about the causes of asthma, we need to think about two things: what made you develop asthma in the first place and, once asthma is established, what factors can set it off.

The reason why you developed asthma in the first place is that you come from a family which has a tendency to develop allergies. This inherited tendency to allergies is called *atopy*, and is discussed in more detail in the first section of this chapter. Asthma does seem to be – at least in part – an inherited condition. Having inherited this tendency, something then happened to you that turned this predisposition into actual asthma; you will find some suggestions as to what this 'something' might have been in the answer to the next question.

The factors that can set off your symptoms or cause you to have an acute asthma attack are usually referred to as 'triggers'. Your own triggers will be unique to you, but the more common ones are discussed in the section 'Triggers' in Chapter 2. It is worth trying to find out what your triggers are, because some of them may be things that you can avoid, and you may therefore be able to reduce your day-to-day symptoms and even limit the number of asthma attacks you have.

I have asthma, which my doctor says is caused by stress. Does stress encourage the development of allergies?

There is little doubt that how we feel can influence our day-to-day health, although this is not the same as saying that an illness or disorder is caused by stress. I suspect that your doctor meant that stress might trigger your asthma attacks. A number of different emotional factors can trigger attacks in people with asthma, and therefore asthma can be more apparent in a person suffering high stress levels. However, the asthma has not been caused in the first place by stress, and it is not more common in people leading stressful lives (there is more information about the causes of asthma in Chapter 2).

What is true of asthma is also true of other allergic diseases. Stress does not cause them but it can trigger attacks, and stress certainly makes it more difficult to cope with the symptoms.

INHERITANCE

Why have I developed allergies when my sister hasn't?

Allergies occur because of a mixture of inherited and environmental factors. You were born with a predisposition to having allergies, which you inherited from your parents. This is called *atopy*, and is discussed in more detail in the section 'Allergy explained' at the beginning of this chapter. Exactly which genes we inherit from our parents is largely a matter of chance, so you may have inherited more 'allergy genes' than your sister. (Genes determine the characteristics that we inherit from our parents, and chromosomes are the structures in our body cells that carry the genes.)

Given that you have this genetically determined tendency to develop allergies, environmental factors become important. The way in which you are first exposed to various allergens will determine whether or not you develop allergic problems. If atopic people were never exposed to allergens, they would not develop allergies! The younger you are when you are first exposed to allergens and the greater the amount of allergen you encounter, the more likely you are to develop an allergy. For example, babies born just before or during the pollen season are more likely to develop hay fever and asthma than those born in winter.

Exposure to allergens is not the only important environmental factor. Interesting new evidence suggests that the more colds you catch in the first few years of life, the less likely you are to develop allergic disorders. We are also becoming more aware that there are other factors, called *adjuvant factors*, that can increase an individual's risk of developing allergies. These adjuvant factors include chemical air pollution and cigarette smoke. For example, babies born to mothers who smoke are twice as likely as other babies to develop asthma.

Once you have an allergy, there are a number of environmental factors, known as *co-factors*, which may – in some people – make their symptoms more severe. These include exercise, aspirin, cold air, fevers and certain foodstuffs.

You can see that not all the children in an atopic family will go on to develop allergies. At present it is difficult to predict who will and who won't, although this will become more possible as we learn more about the genetics of asthma.

Allergies, although more common in childhood and early adulthood, can develop at any time of life, even in old age, so your sister can't yet be certain that she has escaped completely.

Both of my children had eczema as small babies, developed asthma at around 4 years old, and started getting hay fever before they were 10. Are all these problems related, and why don't they all start at the same time? Has one caused the others?

The three problems you describe are related in that they are all allergic disorders that occur in atopic people, and they seem to be linked in the way in which they are inherited. Some individuals (like your children) suffer from all three, others from just one or two.

No one really understands why it is that eczema occurs most commonly in babies, why asthma can appear at any age but does so most commonly in childhood, nor why hay fever is uncommon before a child is 7 years old (the relative incidence of these allergic disorders is shown in Figure 1). However, doctors often see this pattern of eczema being followed by asthma and then hay fever. An infant with eczema has a 50% chance of developing another form of allergic disorder before the age of 10 years. One problem does not cause the other as such (although untreated hay fever can make asthma worse) but they are three related conditions that can occur in the same individual.

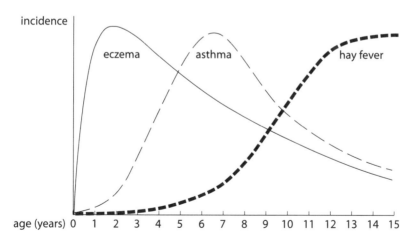

Figure 1 Incidence of eczema, asthma and hay fever at different ages

Your question underlines the limitations of our current knowledge about exactly why particular allergies affect particular people at particular times in their lives. Scientists are currently identifying the genes on the chromosomes that cause people to inherit the tendency to develop allergies. In the future this genetic research may provide a more specific answer to your questions.

THE SCALE OF THE PROBLEM

When I was at school we had never heard of allergy. Now almost every child in my son's class seems to have asthma or an allergy of some kind. Are allergies more common these days?

It is not easy to know exactly how many people suffer from allergies, because many of them never go to their doctor with their problem. Because of this, it is difficult to tell whether allergies really are becoming more common. However, there has been a small number of careful research studies into the prevalence of allergy (the number of people in the population suffering from allergy problems at any one time). These studies have been carried out across a number of years, and have shown fairly conclusively that allergies are indeed becoming more common. Certainly most people's experience, like your own, would seem to agree with this.

Exactly how common are allergy problems?

This is a difficult question to answer, because a large number of people with allergies are never identified and many people who do know that they suffer from allergies never go to their doctor for help because they think their symptoms are too trivial. It is therefore difficult to estimate the true figure, but it is thought that one in three people (that's 18 million of us) suffer from an allergy of some kind in the UK, where we have one of the highest rates of allergic disease in the world. One in 7 school-aged children have asthma, as do one in

10 adults. One in 5 of us will have hay fever at some stage of our lives. Food allergy to peanut alone now affects one in 70 children. Hospital admissions for anaphylaxis, the most severe form of allergic reaction, have increased seven-fold over the past ten years. It is becoming unusual to find a household in the UK where there is not at least one person who suffers from allergy problems. The story is similar in all Westernised countries, although the prevalence of allergic diseases varies considerably in different parts of the world, being much lower in Third World and developing countries.

What are the most common diseases caused by allergy?

Allergy to plant pollens causing hay fever, or seasonal allergic rhinitis (rhinitis is inflammation of the lining of the nose), is probably the most common allergy, affecting about 20% of the population. Asthma is becoming increasingly common, and currently about 15% of all children and 10% of adults are affected.

I know that hay fever is a problem caused by being allergic to pollen, but what other conditions are associated with allergy?

Quite a few different medical problems are at least partly caused by allergy, and these include asthma, hay fever, food allergies, drug allergies, eczema, dermatitis, urticaria (hives and nettle rash), angioedema and anaphylaxis. These are all discussed in other chapters of this book.

2 | Asthma

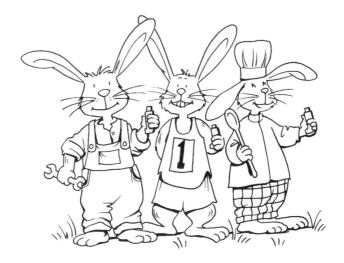

Asthma is not new: it was described by the Chinese before 1000 BC, and was well known to the ancient Greeks. What is new is how asthma appears to be becoming more common – over the past 60 years it has become one of the most important health problems in the Western world. In the UK almost 3 million people suffer from asthma, which means that at least one adult in every 10 has asthma, and at least one in every 7 children. Asthma is now the commonest chronic childhood medical condition, causing more school days to be lost than any other illness. The cost to the economy is enormous: it has been estimated that the financial burden of allergic disease on the National Health Service in primary care alone (excluding hospital services), is £900 million each year. The cost of asthma to the NHS, the Department for Work and Pensions and employers is in excess of £750 million per year.

As modern medicine is seemingly so advanced and asthma now so common, you might think that its diagnosis and treatment would be easy. Unfortunately, this is not always so. The symptoms of asthma can be very variable, and asthma can show itself in a number of different ways. It is not an exaggeration to say that everyone who has asthma is unique. Asthma symptoms can vary not just between individuals but also in the same person on different occasions. This is, in part, because there are so many factors that can bring on the symptoms of asthma, and each factor can produce a different result. This is why it is so important that you understand the whys and wherefores of *your* asthma, and learn not just how to treat your symptoms but also how to prevent them. With this knowledge will come the confidence that you can manage your asthma, which should make every aspect of your life more enjoyable.

ASTHMA EXPLAINED

I have asthma, but no one has ever had the time to tell me exactly what is going on inside my lungs or why I sometimes have difficulty breathing. Please could you explain it to me?

As you know already, asthma is a condition that makes it difficult to move air in and out of your lungs as you breathe. This happens because your airways (the branching tubes leading to and from the lungs' air sacs) are inflamed. This inflammation makes your airways irritable, swollen, red and sore. There are three reasons why this makes your airways narrower:

- The walls of the inflamed airways are swollen and this reduces the size of the air passages inside.

- The inflamed airways produce more mucus and phlegm, which obstructs the air passages.

- The inflamed airways are irritable, and this makes the muscles in the airway wall twitchy and more likely to go into spasm.

The airways of people with asthma are always slightly inflamed, even when they feel well, and this makes it easier for various trigger factors such as allergens, exercise or virus infections to set off an asthma attack. (There is a section on triggers later in this chapter.)

Why does asthma start?

Asthma is a condition that has lots of different causes, and each person's asthma is due to a mixture of these. They can be divided up into hereditary and environmental factors – that is to say, what you have inherited from your parents and what is going on in the world around you.

We know that a predisposition to developing asthma is inherited, so it is a condition that often runs in families. Scientists are beginning to locate the many different genes on our chromosomes that pass on this asthma tendency from one generation to another (genes determine the characteristics that we inherit from our parents, and chromosomes are the structures in our body cells that carry the genes). In the long term, this research may help us to develop better treatments for asthma, and maybe even a cure.

The environmental factors that unmask this predisposition to asthma in a particular individual are difficult to identify. However, we know that if a young baby, or even a fetus before it is born, is exposed to high levels of certain allergens (e.g. pollen or the house dust mite), that child will be more likely to develop asthma later in life.

So, things that may have made your inherited tendency more likely to develop into actual asthma include:

- being brought up in a home where there was a pet, especially a cat;

- if foods such as cow's milk and eggs were introduced into your diet too early;

- if you were born at a time of year when the pollen count was high;

- if you received frequent courses of antibiotics in early life;

- if you were protected from common infections such as colds and gastroenteritis by not mixing with groups of other children.

There are other factors, called *adjuvant factors*, that can also increase your chances of getting asthma. These adjuvant factors include chemical air pollution and cigarette smoke. Babies born to mothers who smoke are twice as likely as other babies to develop asthma at some stage in their lives.

This may help to explain why you have developed asthma but perhaps your brothers and sisters have not. It is not just a simple matter of inheritance, and it can be a difficult task to predict which family members will develop it – one that is made more difficult because there is no fixed age at which asthma starts. Although two-thirds of people with asthma first get their symptoms in childhood, it can develop at any time of life, even when people are in their sixties or seventies.

Why don't I have asthma all of the time?

One of the hallmarks of asthma is that its symptoms vary a great deal from day to day and also over longer periods of time. You may have periods of your life when your asthma is virtually trouble-free. Similarly, you might find that even when your asthma is causing you problems, you have good days and bad days, or even good weeks and bad weeks.

Sometimes we can see the reason for this variation. For example, you may find that your asthma is less troublesome when you are on holiday and less stressed. On the other hand, you may find that there are particular times of the year when your asthma is worse because of a particular type of pollen or changes in the weather. Some people's asthma is much worse when they have a cold, and better in between colds. In women, asthma symptoms can vary with their menstrual cycle.

How you take your treatment will also affect your symptoms. When you take the right preventative treatment regularly, your asthma symptoms should be well controlled, but if you are not yet on the correct treatment or you don't take it regularly, it is going to be much less effective.

Sometimes there is no obvious reason for the variations in your asthma symptoms. They just happen.

Asthma seems to be getting so much more common. Why is this?

You're right; asthma is getting more common. Even when you take into account the fact that both doctors and the general public are more aware of asthma as a condition (which means that milder cases that in the past might have been ignored are now being correctly diagnosed), there is no doubt that the number of people with asthma has been increasing steadily for the last 40 years.

If we think about genetic factors, it is unlikely that there has been a major change in the way that asthma is inherited during this relatively short time, so we suspect that the reason for the increase is something to do with our environment. Increasing levels of air pollution, our modern diet with its high level of processed foods lacking in vitamins, our central-heated, double-glazed buildings with their high levels of house dust mite, and many other things about our modern day lifestyle might be responsible. There is a great deal of research being carried out at present on this subject, as asthma imposes a major social and financial burden on most industrialised countries of the world.

Are there any differences between asthma in males and in females?

Yes, there are quite marked differences. Although the different roles of men and women in our society are rapidly changing, it is still true that men are more likely to work outside the home, and women within it. The different triggers for asthma that men and women encounter will therefore vary according to their environment. There are other differences: men seem to be more likely to deny their asthma and to be reluctant to seek diagnosis and treatment. Women may experience additional problems with their asthma during their menstrual periods. Other lifestyle factors such as smoking habits, participation in sport and exposure to certain chemicals vary between the sexes.

There also seems to be a difference between males and females in the way that asthma behaves throughout life. In children under the age of 7, asthma is almost twice as common in boys as it is in girls. This seems to be because boy babies, although on average heavier and longer than girl babies, are born with smaller airways, which are more prone to being affected by asthma. As boy children grow older, their airways become larger and they are more likely than girls to 'grow out of' their asthma and to become symptom-free. By the late teens, asthma is equally common in both sexes and by the twenties it is slightly more common in women and remains so throughout the later years.

I'm fed up with having to take medications every day. Can't asthma be cured?

No, it cannot be cured at present. The outlook isn't all gloomy though, as quite a large number of people with asthma seem to develop symptom-free periods at some stage in their lives. Unfortunately, they cannot be said to have grown out of their asthma, because the symptoms often come back again.

A number of ways of curing asthma are currently being researched. These include how to switch asthma off in people who have already developed it, and techniques for preventing it from developing in the first place (see Chapter 11, 'The Future').

Perhaps you would be a suitable candidate for immunotherapy (allergen desensitisation, see Chapter 1). Although this is time-consuming, as it involves trips to hospital for injections – initially once or twice a week, reducing to monthly after a few months – it could reduce or eliminate your need for regular drug treatment. However, it is offered to only a limited number of people because of the shortage of allergy specialists in the UK.

In the meantime, take steps to reduce the impact of asthma on your life. Get the best treatment available – your goal should be to live as normal a life as possible with as few symptoms and side effects as possible. It sounds as if you find your treatment difficult to take. Why not go and talk to your doctor and ask about alternative medications? There are now some asthma drugs that can be taken in tablet form that might be suitable for you, and there may be ways that your doctor can simplify your treatment regimen.

SYMPTOMS

My daughter and I both have asthma, but you would hardly know we had the same problem as our symptoms are so different. Is this unusual?

Not at all! Everyone who has asthma is unique, each person having their own pattern and type of symptoms and a different set of trigger factors (there is a section on triggers later in this chapter). Although health-care professionals can be expert in their knowledge of asthma in general, you are your own expert on your particular type of asthma. The more aware and better informed you are about it, the better you will be able to control your symptoms.

What are the typical symptoms of asthma?

It's not easy to answer this question, as there are so many different ways in which asthma can show itself, and it can even be different in the same person at different times. The symptoms that occur most commonly are those of wheeze, cough and shortness of breath. These are often worse at night and first thing on waking in the morning. Symptoms are also commonly triggered by exercise, allergen exposure, viral infections, cold air, cigarette smoke and chemical fumes. Sometimes, laughing and crying can bring symptoms on. One of the hallmarks of asthma is that the symptoms vary over time, being different at different times of day and also from day to day. Some doctors used to believe that people could only be diagnosed as having asthma if they wheezed, but we now realise that sometimes cough is the main symptom, especially in children.

As well as different symptoms there can be different patterns of asthma. Some people with asthma have symptoms almost every day; others have their symptoms in the form of acute attacks, and are well in between attacks.

I sometimes find it hard to judge how bad my asthma is. What symptoms mean I'm having a bad attack?

This is a very common problem. People who have had asthma for a while may get used to having narrowed airways, and begin to consider this normal. This makes them under-estimate how bad their asthma is at any one time, and leads to dangerous delays in seeking medical help when things get worse. This is where measurement of your lung function with a small device called a peak flow meter (peak flow measurements are discussed in the section 'Diagnosis and assessment' later in this chapter) can be very helpful, as it gives an objective measure of asthma severity.

Obviously I don't know the details of your asthma and the problems it causes you, so I have to answer this question in general terms. Bearing this in mind, below are the warning signs that should signal that your attack is a severe one:

- Symptoms that are unusually severe or unusually prolonged for you.

- Unusual symptoms that you have not had before.

- Breathlessness that is so bad that you find it hard to use your normal inhalers properly.

- Breathlessness that is so bad that you find it difficult to speak.

- Symptoms that are not relieved by your usual reliever medication.

- Only short-lived (less than 4 hours) improvement from your usual reliever medication.

- A very fast heart rate (this can be felt at the wrist or at the neck) – i.e. more than 120 beats per minute in an adult and more than 140 beats per minute in a child.

- A drop in your peak flow measurements to less than half of your usual level.

- Feeling exhausted by the effort to breathe.

- Any degree of blueness around your lips or of your tongue.

Asthma attacks can come on at any time, and they can be severe from the start. Mild attacks can develop into severe ones, and this can last anything from just a few minutes to several days. Asthma does not conform to a set pattern, and so it is really important that you take notice of any worsening of your symptoms. Always carry your reliever medication with you, use it when you feel your symptoms coming on, and get medical help if your reliever treatment does not produce a lasting improvement or if you have any of the other warning signs listed above.

TRIGGERS

What does my doctor mean when he talks about triggers of my asthma?

A trigger is anything that acts to make your asthma worse, either by causing increased symptoms or by bringing on an asthma attack. Not all people with asthma have the same trigger factors, and so something that causes you frequent problems might have no effect on someone else.

You may not know all of the triggers that affect your asthma. Some are obvious, others less so. You can read more about identifying trigger factors in Appendix 1.

The most common triggers are:

- The **common cold virus (upper respiratory tract infections)** Most people's asthma gets worse when they develop a cold. This is particularly true in children, for whom this might be the only trigger. Often the symptoms of asthma persist after the cold itself has gone, sometimes for as long as six weeks.

- **Allergens** Exposure to allergens such as cat or dog fur, house dust mites, pollen and mould spores is a frequent cause of asthma symptoms and acute attacks. People with asthma are particularly troubled by these allergens when they also have a cold.

- **Exercise** Coughing and wheezing brought on by exercise are very common in people with asthma. Exercise can be a particularly potent trigger factor when the air is cold and dry.

- **Emotion** Laughing, crying, getting excited or being upset can all trigger an asthma attack. This is particularly so in small children.

- **Cold air** Changes in air temperature, particularly going from a warm environment into cold air, can bring on symptoms.

- **Air pollution** Traffic fumes, industrial waste products, aerosol fumes and cigarette smoke can all be potent triggers for asthma.

- **Occupation** Substances that are encountered in the work environment can become triggers for asthma.

- **Drugs** Certain drugs can trigger asthma attacks in some people. The commonest of these are aspirin, anti-inflammatory painkillers such as ibuprofen (brand names include Brufen, Nurofen and Cuprofen), and two classes of drugs, beta-blockers and angiotensin-converting enzyme (ACE) inhibitors, both used for the treatment of high blood pressure. Once a problem with any of these drugs has been diagnosed, the drug in question should always be avoided; there are alternatives that are just as effective.

- **Foods** It is a common misconception that foodstuffs such as milk products or preservatives are frequent triggers for asthma. In fact, it is relatively unusual for them to have this effect. There is no doubt that food allergies exist, but they tend to cause other allergic problems such as eczema or urticaria (both discussed in Chapter 3), and are rarely responsible for triggering asthma. An exception is sulphites, found in dried fruits, wine and shellfish. Even if a food has been definitely identified as a trigger factor, it is important to remember that it is unlikely to be the only trigger involved. Although it would be sensible to avoid the food responsible wherever possible, you will probably need to use asthma medications as well to control your symptoms.

Why does other people's cigarette smoke make my asthma worse? I don't smoke.

Cigarette smoke is a complicated cocktail full of different chemicals and gases, many of which are very irritant to the lungs. Passive smoking (breathing in other people's cigarette smoke) can be irritating even to the lungs of people who do not have asthma, making them cough and feel tight-chested. In asthma the lungs are always inflamed, and are therefore more vulnerable to the effects of the smoke. It is likely to make you cough and wheeze, and the more inflamed your lungs are, the greater the chance that the smoke will aggravate your asthma.

My asthma seems to behave differently at different times of year, and I think this is to do with changes in the weather. Is this possible?

Yes, it is possible, as changes in the weather can affect your asthma in two ways. Firstly, changes in air temperature and humidity are both factors that can bring on asthma symptoms. This will be most noticeable when the air temperature changes from warm to cold, and when the air is particularly dry or particularly wet and misty. Many people find that spring and autumn are the times when the weather seems to affect them the most.

Secondly, the weather affects the level and the distribution of allergens that can trigger asthma, such as pollens, moulds and spores, and the house dust mite. The house dust mite and moulds thrive in warm, damp conditions, and are therefore likely to be particularly troublesome in the autumn. The pollen count (explained in the section 'Pollens' in Chapter 9) tends to be highest in the summer, on days when the air is hot and still.

I have asthma and am keen not to do anything that might make it worse. Are there any sports or hobbies I should avoid because they could trigger my symptoms?

My aim in treating people with asthma is to enable them to lead full lives and take part in all the activities that they find enjoyable. There are, however, certain activities that are more likely than others to bring on asthma.

Hobbies that involve fumes and dust, such as model building and certain forms of DIY, might trigger your asthma. Any activity that brings you into contact with animals, especially ones with fur or hair, could also affect you if you develop an allergy to them.

When it comes to sports, it is worth remembering that many top athletes have asthma. Sport is less likely to bring on your symptoms if it takes place in the warm (either during the summer or indoors), if the air is humid (such as in a swimming pool), if you perform warm-up exercises beforehand, and if the sport involves a steady level of activity. Sports that involve sudden bursts of vigorous exercise, especially if played outdoors in winter, might be more of a problem. However, if you find that you experience asthma symptoms because of exercise, these can be much reduced (or even abolished altogether) by performing warm-up exercises and by taking two puffs of your reliever (blue) inhaler approximately 15 minutes before you start. This is a much better option than waiting until you become breathless before you use your reliever inhaler: be pro-active rather than reactive.

Exercise and contact with cats and horses all make my asthma worse. Can I make myself more resistant to these triggers?

Your general health is important in asthma. If you keep yourself fit, eat well, have enough sleep and reduce the stress levels in your life as far as possible, you are likely to be more resistant to the effects of your trigger factors. However, healthy living alone is unlikely to prevent all your symptoms, and it is therefore vital that you take other measures to control your asthma.

First and foremost, you should treat the inflammation in your airways (the underlying problem in all asthma) by using – on a regular basis – adequate levels of your preventer medications as prescribed by your doctor.

Secondly, you should reduce your exposure to things that are known to make the inflammation of your airways worse, such as environmental allergens, air pollution and cigarette smoke. (Chapter 9 offers some suggestions for ways to avoid common allergens and other triggers.) Because you are allergic to cats, it is not a good idea to have a pet cat yourself; every part of your home, including your bedding and your clothes, would soon become covered in the very potent allergen a cat produces, which is found in its skin scales, saliva and urine. This would be sure to provoke your asthma symptoms. However, if you are to visit a home with a cat or want to go horse-riding, you could try taking two puffs of your reliever inhaler 15 minutes beforehand, as this may protect you to some extent. Remember to change your clothes when you get home and put them straight in the wash, as they will carry a hefty dose of allergen, which mustn't be spread around your home.

Don't avoid exercise, as it is an important part of maintaining good general health. There are ways in which you can exercise without developing symptoms such as wheeziness (see also the answer above).

Combining these measures will make you less vulnerable to the trigger factors for your asthma, both the ones you know about and those that are less obvious.

I am 18 and have had asthma since I was 4 years old. Are there any particular jobs that I should avoid?

There are certain workplace conditions that are not advisable for anyone with asthma. Dust, fumes, smoke and chemicals are all triggers that are likely to make asthma worse, and should be avoided. Think carefully about what factors tend to trigger your asthma and try to avoid them as far as possible in your place of work. With new legislation, most indoor environments are smoke-free zones, and I would thoroughly recommend anyone with asthma to choose a workplace entirely free of cigarette smoke (the reasons for this were discussed earlier in this section).

Since a change in the law in October 2004, people with asthma are included within the Disability Discrimination Act of 1995, and are no longer automatically banned from joining the police force or fire service. Each candidate is now assessed on an individual basis. The ambulance service employs people with asthma provided that they don't contravene any of the Group 2 DVLA requirements for driving. In particular, they must not have 'any condition which causes any daytime/awake time sleepiness', so someone with asthma that frequently disturbs their sleep would not be considered.

The Army and the Royal Navy will not accept anyone who has asthma at the time of applying, but may consider you if you have neither needed nor received any anti-asthma treatment in the previous four years. You will have to be assessed by an armed services medical specialist, and be aware that if you are found to have hidden any relevant information you could be dismissed.

The Royal Air Force does not accept potential candidates if they have ever had asthma.

If you have asthma you may have greater problems when scuba-diving because of the triggers you are exposed to when you dive (cold dry air, exercise, stress, emotion), and even though you may be allowed to dive recreationally if your asthma is well controlled (see Chapter 8), you would not be accepted as a commercial diver.

My asthma has got a lot worse since I changed jobs. I know it's not stress-related, because I'm far more relaxed now than I was before in my previous work. Can you think of any other reasons why this has happened?

Working in a new job can exacerbate asthma in someone who already has it, or even cause asthma in someone who has never had it before. I don't know what your job is, but you might now be experiencing a greater exposure to one or more of the trigger factors that make your asthma worse. For example, you might have to work in a smoky office instead of a smoke-free one, or there might be higher pollen levels in the area where you now work, or the nature of your work might mean that you are now exposed to a large number of other people's respiratory viruses – for example, if you are a school teacher or if you work in a large open-plan office.

There is also a type of asthma, called *occupational asthma*, that is directly caused by exposure to particular substances found in the workplace. These substances include:

- metals, including nickel, cobalt and aluminium;
- vegetable dusts such as coffee, grains and flour;
- animals and insects;
- polyurethane, spray paints and epoxy resins;
- soldering flux;
- wood dusts;
- dust from latex rubber.

This list is not exhaustive, but the Department of Health (address in Appendix 2) can supply more information about occupational triggers. Anyone who has developed asthma after starting a particular job and who suspects that a substance in the workplace may be responsible should ask to be referred to an occupational health specialist. The Health and Safety Executive (address also in Appendix 2) can help you, and you may be eligible for industrial compensation. It is important to decide whether you are suffering from occupational asthma, as further exposure to an occupational trigger factor could lead to permanent lung damage, whereas protecting you from the substance in question might result in a great improvement in your asthma. The first step is to look at the pattern of your asthma symptoms and to see whether they are worse during the working week (either at or after work) and improve when you have time off work.

There is more information about occupational asthma and other workplace allergies in Chapter 7.

DIAGNOSIS AND ASSESSMENT

How do doctors and nurses diagnose asthma if it can be so different in different people?

If you came to consult me, the first very important step that I would take in making a diagnosis of asthma would be to spend as much time as possible in talking to you so that I was able to develop a clear picture about what symptoms you have, when they occur, what triggers them and what makes them better. I would also want to ask you about other members of your family who have had problems with related atopic disorders: not only asthma but also eczema, hay fever, perennial allergic rhinitis and urticaria (all these are discussed elsewhere in this book). I would also ask questions about your home and your work, to see if there were trigger factors there that might be important, and find out what medications you have been taking.

I would then examine you, firstly to look specifically for clues to asthma (e.g. a change in the shape of your chest, wheezing when I listen with a stethoscope, and whether you have eczema) and secondly to make sure that there was no suggestion of other problems that could be confused with asthma.

Usually by this stage it would be fairly clear whether or not you have asthma. However, it might still be useful for me to perform a

number of different tests that would give me additional helpful information (there is no single test that can diagnose asthma, so we
combine information from several). These include tests of how well
your lungs are working (both peak flow measurement and more
sophisticated lung function testing), skin-prick testing for diagnosing
allergies, and perhaps a blood test to look for evidence of allergy (all
these tests are explained in detail in Appendix 1). In children I would
also measure height and weight so that I could assess their growth.

A particularly useful test measures your response to a dose of bronchodilator medication such as salbutamol (e.g. Ventolin and Airomir)
which will open up your airways if they are tight because of asthma.
A small device called a peak flow meter (there is more about these
meters later in this section) is used to measure how hard you can
blow before, and then 15 minutes after, a dose of salbutamol. If you
have asthma but are not taking anti-asthma medications, an
improvement of at least 20% should be seen. This improvement does
not occur in people who do not have asthma, nor in people with chest
problems due to other causes.

It might be that, despite doing everything I have described, it
would still not be possible to decide whether you have asthma. In this
case, the best option would be to treat you with effective anti-asthma
medication whilst monitoring your symptoms and peak flow recordings, using a record card. We would need to continue this for four
weeks, because it takes this long for the medication to make a difference to your lung function. If I saw a significant improvement over
this time, you would almost certainly have asthma, and you would
need to continue taking the treatment.

*My son, aged 18 months, has a terrible cough, and my GP says it
is asthma and has prescribed some treatment. I thought asthma
made you wheeze. How does he know this is asthma?*

Asthma is different in every individual, and different people
experience a different combination of the common symptoms
of wheeze, cough, shortness of breath and difficulty in breathing.

In children, it is relatively common for asthma to produce coughing without wheezing. Your GP has probably asked you questions about your son's cough, including, among many others, at what time of the day and night it is worse, and what triggers tend to bring it on. It is from this information that he would have made the diagnosis of asthma. If the cough is made better by the anti-asthma medications your GP has prescribed, this is final proof that your son has asthma.

I think that my asthma has been brought on by being exposed to paint fumes at work. How do doctors diagnose occupational asthma?

To be able to diagnose you as having occupational asthma, two things are necessary. Firstly we have to identify a particular chemical or allergen in your workplace that is known to cause occupational asthma. Certain paints and thinners fall into this category. Secondly we would have to demonstrate that your asthma is worse while you are working but better at weekends and during holidays taken away from your workplace. Monitoring your symptoms and lung function using a peak flow meter can help to do this. Final proof that your asthma is occupational can be obtained by protecting you from contact with the agent responsible and showing that your asthma has improved.

There is more information about occupational asthma in Chapter 7.

I don't find it easy to tell how bad my asthma is. On days that I think I'm fine, my doctor says my chest is really tight. Is there a way that I can assess my asthma?

The simplest way of assessing your asthma is by noting how often your symptoms occur and how bad they are. This is often done with the help of a symptom score card or diary. By doing this, you will see when your symptoms occur, and you may be able to recognise a particular pattern (women may find their symptoms follow

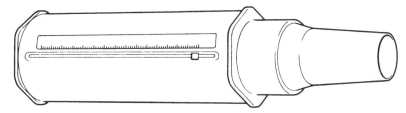

Figure 2 Peak flow meter
(Courtesy of Education for Health)

their menstrual cycle), or relate them to particular triggers such as colds or exposure to cigarette smoke. However, some people find that they are not very good at recognising their symptoms, and it sounds as if you may be one of these.

Another way of assessing your asthma is by measuring your peak expiratory flow. This is a measurement of how hard you can blow, and is measured by using a small portable device called a peak flow meter (shown in Figure 2). Although there are charts that tell you what a 'normal' result is for someone of your age, sex and height, it is more useful to get a feel for your own personal normal level by making measurements when you are well. A reduction in your peak flow recording below this level tells you that the control of your asthma is not as good as it might be, and that you should either increase your treatment (if you have already agreed this with your doctor) or see your doctor as soon as possible.

My GP has given me a peak flow meter and has shown me how to blow into it, but I am not sure how often I should use it nor what to look out for. Can you help?

Peak flow meters are used to measure the volume (the amount) of air that you can blow out from your lungs each second (i.e. the air flow). In asthma, the flow from the lungs is reduced because the airways are narrowed. Measuring your peak flow is therefore a way of measuring how much your asthma is affecting your lungs; the higher the recording, the better your lungs are functioning. Also, peak flow measurements in asthma vary from day to day – a lot more than in people who don't have asthma. This variation becomes less once the asthma is properly treated, so it is a useful way of assessing the effectiveness of your treatment.

Different people use peak flow meters in different ways. Some like to measure their peak flow every day, as a check on how well their lungs are functioning. This can be particularly useful for people who have got so used to their symptoms that they sometimes fail to notice that their asthma is getting worse. A drop in their peak flow alerts them to the fact that they need to take action.

Others prefer to use their peak flow meter as a tool to help them assess their asthma on the days when they are not feeling so good. On these days, measurement of peak flow can help to assess the severity of an attack, and can guide you in deciding what action to take.

Peak flow meters can also be used to assess how effective a change in treatment is. If your doctor suggests an alteration to your medication, you can monitor what benefits, if any, this brings by measuring your peak flow for four weeks after the change is made. If the change is effective, you will see a gradual increase in your peak flow over this time and a reduction in its variability.

In your case, I don't know how long you have had asthma, nor how bad it is. However, I would suggest that you might find it useful to measure your peak flow morning and evening on a daily basis for a period of about a month, so that you get a feel for what your 'normal' values are. You will probably find that your peak flow is slightly lower in the morning than in the evening. This variation, called *diurnal variation*, happens because your lungs are often a little tight on waking. This wears off during the day. Once you have a good idea of what is normal for you, you can use your peak flow meter as a way of assessing your lungs on days that you feel under par.

Trouble signs to look out for are:

- your peak flow recordings are dropping, or are below your normal level;

- there is an increasing difference between your morning and your evening peak flow readings, with lower recordings in the mornings;

- there is an increasing variation between readings, with unusually low recordings on some days.

If you notice any of these, see your doctor as soon as possible, and consider increasing your treatment in the meantime.

TREATMENT

I am a teacher in a secondary school and I get very confused about all the different types of inhaler used by my pupils for their asthma. What's in all these different devices? Do they all work the same way?

Inhalers are the most efficient way of giving asthma medications, as the drug is delivered directly to the place they are needed (the lungs) by breathing them in. The drugs work more quickly when inhaled than medications taken by mouth and much smaller amounts are needed to produce the same results, which in turn reduces the likelihood of side effects. Even small children are rarely prescribed medications to take by mouth because, with the newer inhaler devices available, even a baby can take medications by inhalation.

As you say, there are many different devices available (there is more information about them in the answer to the next question), and each type requires a different level of co-ordination to use it correctly. There are also several different types of medication that may be prescribed. Each drug may (if its patent has expired) be manufactured by several different companies, and each drug has two names – the *generic* name, which is the pharmacological name (spelled with a small letter), and the *trade* name (spelled with a capital letter), which is chosen by the individual drug company. The particular medication and delivery device that suits one child will not necessarily suit another, hence the range you see among your pupils.

Broadly speaking, medications for the treatment of asthma can be divided into two groups, which we call *preventers* and *relievers*. The colour of the inhaler will give you some idea of which type of drug it contains: preventer inhalers are usually beige, brown, orange or maroon; reliever inhalers are usually blue; and long-acting reliever inhalers are usually green. This list is not complete, as other colours are used by some pharmaceutical companies, but you will find it useful as a rough guide.

Preventers
Preventer medications treat the inflammation found in the airways in asthma, and are used, as the name implies, to prevent the symptoms of asthma and asthma attacks. To do this, these medications need to be used regularly every day, even during periods when there are no symptoms. The doctor can adjust the dose of the preventer medication according to need. Preventers do not work immediately, but instead act over a period of time to treat the inflammation and stabilise the asthma. They will have no effect in the case of an acute attack. Most preventers are taken by being inhaled; because they are taken on a twice-daily basis, most children will keep their preventer medication at home.

The most commonly prescribed preventers are the inhaled steroids, which include beclometasone, budesonide and fluticasone. Another type of anti-inflammatory drug is the cromones (sodium cromoglicate and nedocromil sodium) – these are less commonly prescribed as they are less effective than inhaled steroids.

Relievers
Reliever medications (bronchodilators) fall into two groups: short-acting and long-acting relievers.

Short-acting bronchodilators relieve asthma symptoms by relaxing and opening up (dilating) the airways, and should be used only when symptoms occur or before exercise. They act quickly and effectively, relieving asthma symptoms within 15 minutes and lasting about 4 hours. They have no long-term beneficial effect on asthma, as they do not reduce the amount of inflammation in the lungs, and should be used only when needed, because taking them too frequently can make the lungs less responsive to them. The most commonly used drugs are ipratropium bromide, salbutamol and terbutaline.

Long-acting bronchodilators last approximately 12 hours, and are used in people who are already on regular preventer medications and who need to use frequent doses of their short-acting bronchodilator. These include formoterol and salmeterol.

Some inhalers contain a combination of two different drugs (a preventer and a long-acting reliever) for use by people who use both types of medication and find it more convenient to use a single inhaler.

Children with asthma need free access to their reliever medication at all times, because delay in taking this treatment could allow symptoms to develop into a severe asthma attack.

If you would like more information about how asthma affects children at school, contact Asthma UK (details in Appendix 2) and ask for a school information pack.

I'm not very happy with the inhalers I have for my asthma, as I find them difficult to use. What can I do?

You don't say which type of inhaler you are using but, as you are finding it difficult to use, I suspect that it is a metered dose inhaler (shown in Figure 3). This is the most commonly used type of inhaler, and most asthma treatments are available in this form. However, it does have disadvantages, the most important one being that it can be difficult to use because very good co-ordination is needed to use it correctly.

I suggest that you go back to your GP's surgery or health centre and ask for an appointment in their asthma clinic – this is usually run by a practice nurse. Some extra training in how to use your current inhaler correctly may be the answer to your problem, or it may turn out that you would be better off with a different device altogether.

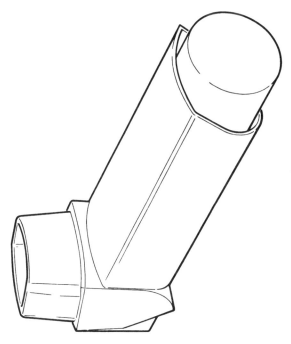

Figure 3 Metered dose inhaler
(Courtesy of Education for Health)

There are over a dozen different types of inhaler now available, and these various devices all have their own advantages and disadvantages. Some are much easier to use than others. They fall into the following categories:

- metered dose inhalers
- breath-activated metered dose inhalers
- dry powder devices
- spacer devices
- nebulisers

What suits one person will not necessarily suit another, and your doctor or nurse will be able to help you choose the one that suits you best and to show you how to use it. The following descriptions will give you an idea of the range available.

- The **metered dose inhaler** (available for beclometasone, budesonide, ipratropium, nedocromil, salbutamol, salbutamol + ipratropium, salmeterol, sodium cromoglicate; also available in a CFC-free form for beclometasone, ciclesonide, fluticasone, fluticasone + salmeterol, nedocromil, salbutamol + salmeterol).

  This device releases a fine aerosol of the active ingredient, propelled by a harmless gas. The spray comes out very quickly and, unless you breathe in at exactly the same time that the spray is released, and at a rate similar to that at which the spray travels, a lot of it will hit the back of your throat and not enough of the drug will be delivered to the lungs. The result of this is that you will get little benefit from the inhaler, and you may get unpleasant problems in your mouth and throat (details are given later in this chapter). The casing of the inhaler is a different colour for each medication. Figure 3 shows a typical metered dose inhaler.

- **Breath-activated metered dose inhalers**. There are two of these:

  - the Autohaler (Figure 4) – available for beclometasone (previously known as beclomethasone);

  - the Easi-Breathe (Figure 5) – beclometasone, salbutamol and sodium cromoglicate.

  They both contain an aerosol canister similar to a metered dose inhaler but the dose of medicine is released automatically when you breathe in through the mouthpiece. This makes them easier to use correctly, as the puff of medication is always released at the right time and little co-ordination is needed. They are about the same size as a metered dose inhaler, so are convenient to carry.

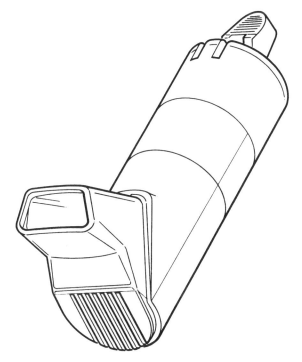

Figure 4 Autohaler
(Courtesy of Education for Health)

- **Dry powder devices.** These include:

  - the Accuhaler – fluticasone, salmeterol, fluticasone + salmeterol, salbutamol;

  - the Diskhaler – beclometasone, fluticasone, salmeterol;

  - the Easyhaler – beclometasone, budesonide, salbutamol;

  - the Clickhaler – beclometasone, salbutamol;

  - the Novolizer – beclometasone;

  - the Pulvinal – beclometasone, salbutamol;

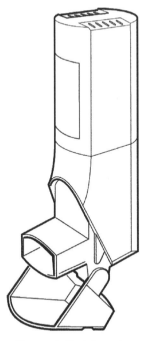

Figure 5 Easi-Breathe
(Courtesy of Education for Health)

- the Turbohaler – budesonide, formoterol, budesonide + formoterol, terbutaline;
- the Twisthaler – mometasone.

In these devices the drugs are in powder form, rather than in the pressurised aerosol form used in metered dose inhalers. Some people find the taste of the powder preferable, but others don't like it and it makes some people cough.. These are all breath-activated and therefore easy to use. You can monitor how many doses of the drug are left in the device either by looking through a clear window to see how much powder remains or by a dose counter, something which is not possible with most metered dose inhalers.

- **Spacer devices**. These are of two types:

  - large-volume spacers, such as the Volumatic and the Nebuhaler;

  - small-volume spacers, such as the Able Spacer, AeroChamber, Nebuchamber, Pocket Chamber.

  These spacer devices fit onto a metered dose inhaler and make it easier to use. (Note that not all inhalers fit into each spacer device.) The inhaler is activated to spray the drug into the spacer, where the aerosolised particles stay until you breathe them in. There is no need to co-ordinate the firing of your inhaler with your breathing, and more of the drug is delivered to your lungs (where it is most needed) rather than perhaps ending up in your mouth. The large devices are too big to fit easily into a pocket or handbag, and are being superseded by the small spacers. Face-masks that fit onto the spacer mouth-piece are available for all spacers. These should be added for pre-school children, and for adults who are using their inhaler when particularly breathless. Figures 6, 7 and 8 show some typical spacer devices.

- **Nebulisers**. A nebuliser is a small chamber that is filled with a liquid form of an asthma medication. A compressor is used to blow air or oxygen through the liquid to make a continuous fine mist that can be inhaled through a mouth-piece or face-mask. Nebulisers are occasionally used to treat severe attacks of asthma at a doctor's surgery or in an accident and emergency (A&E) department. However, research has shown that, for treating most asthma attacks in children and adults, multiple doses of reliever medicine given through a spacer device are at least as effective as a nebuliser.

  Most people with asthma will not need to use a nebuliser at home, because their inhaled medicine is best delivered by an inhaler or by an inhaler with a spacer. Rarely, a person with severe asthma symptoms may need to use a nebuliser for their

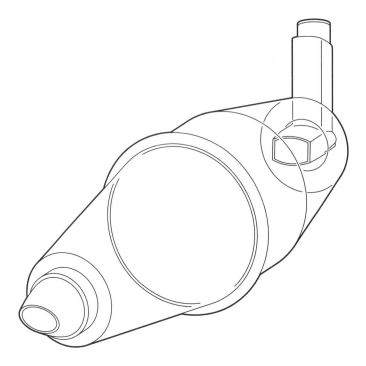

Figure 6 The Volumatic spacer device
(Courtesy of Education for Health)

reliever and preventer medications at home. Nebulisers should only be used under the supervision of your doctor or hospital consultant.

What are the pros and cons of the different types of inhalers?

L et's take them type by type.

Metered dose inhalers used alone can be difficult to use because you need to co-ordinate your breathing with the activation of the aerosol. If most of the spray hits the back of your throat instead of going into your lungs, too little gets to where it is needed, so the

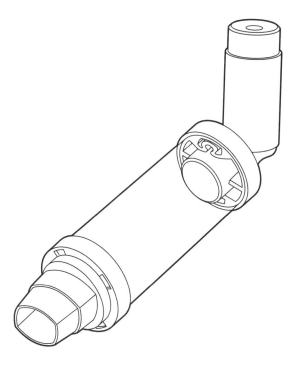

Figure 7 The Aerochamber
(Courtesy of Education for Health)

inhaler fails to work. If the inhaler is a reliever inhaler, you will then have to take repeated doses to get relief of your symptoms, and the drug that is left in your mouth and throat is swallowed and absorbed into the blood-stream. It can then be absorbed into other organs of the body, where it can produce side effects – the most common are tremor (a fine trembling), a fast heart rate, and a feeling of being 'revved up' or anxious. With steroid inhalers (except for ciclesonide), the drug left in the mouth and throat can lead to oral thrush and a hoarse voice.

With most inhalers, there is no accurate way of knowing how many doses are left in the aerosol, so, unless you always carry a spare, there is the risk that it will suddenly run out, leaving you

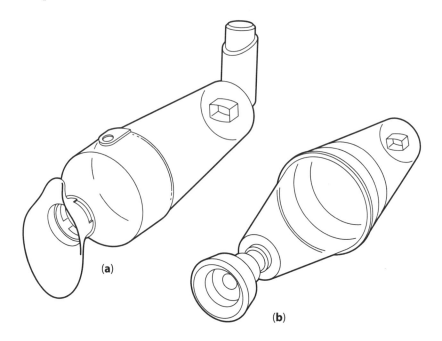

Figure 8 (**a**) The Nebuhaler with Nalato mask
and (**b**) the Volumatic device with Laerdal mask
(Courtesy of Education for Health)

without treatment. Bear in mind that, in an emergency, any pharmacy will let you have a reliever inhaler without a prescription.

On the plus side, these devices are small and easily portable, and
give you a wide choice of treatments, as most asthma medications
come in this format.

Metered dose inhalers with a spacer are much easier to use.
However, they are more bulky to carry around.

Breath-activated metered dose inhalers are easy to use because
the aerosol fires automatically when you breathe in. They are small
and portable. The one main disadvantage is that no one format is
made with the full range of asthma medications you might want to
use, because in general each device is made by only one drug com-

pany. In some circumstances this means you might have to use more than one type of device or change to a different brand of drug.

Dry powder inhalers are easy to use because the powder is released only when you breathe in. They are small and portable, but some contain only a few doses at a time, so you might need to carry spares. Only one device is made with the full range of asthma drugs, so if your doctor decides to change your medication you might need to change to a different device.

Nebulisers are complex pieces of medical equipment and should be used only under the supervision of your doctor. It is vital that the nebuliser is matched correctly to the compressor, and that both are appropriate for the drug to be nebulised. The plastic components need to be replaced frequently, and the compressor serviced regularly. Using a nebuliser is time-consuming, taking 10–15 minutes per medication. They are expensive, cumbersome and heavy to carry around, and need a source of electricity. If you use a nebuliser for a reliever medication when you are wheezy, tight and out of breath, there is a risk that, at first, the nebulisation will make you worse. This is because the mist is cold and when the cold droplets reach your airways they can trigger even more spasm. Because of this, reliever medications should ideally be nebulised using oxygen instead of air.

A better option for most people is to use a metered dose inhaler with a spacer device, and a face-mask if needed, and to take repeated doses if necessary.

Are there any medicines in tablet or liquid form that I can use instead of inhalers?

Although most asthma medication is designed to be taken by inhalation, there are some asthma drugs that are taken by mouth:

- **Leukotriene receptor antagonists** work by blocking the cell receptor for certain chemicals (the leukotrienes) that cause inflammation, and are released during an allergic reaction.

These drugs are not effective in all people, and the only way of finding out if they work for you is by a trial of treatment. They can be used for children as young as 6 months. Your doctor will prescribe these only if you are already taking inhaled steroids as well as a reliever inhaler and your symptoms are still not controlled, although in young children they may be used alone. They can be effective in treating hay fever and perennial rhinitis (see Chapter 4 for more information) as well as asthma; good news if you suffer from both problems.

- **Corticosteroid tablets (prednisolone)** can be used in two ways: to treat an acute severe attack of asthma, when they are given for a short period of time, usually 5 to 14 days (3 days in small children); and, less commonly, as a long-term treatment for severe asthma. The common side effects of short-term treatment with oral steroids (steroids taken by mouth) are indigestion and increased appetite, but there are many more serious side effects of long-term treatment, and people taking them need careful monitoring. If you have taken oral steroids for more than 3 weeks, you must not stop taking this treatment suddenly, as this can be dangerous (there is more information on this later). You will need to reduce the dose of prednisolone slowly, under the supervision of your doctor. You should carry a card, giving details of your medical condition and the steroid dosage.

Does my reliever inhaler medication have any side effects?

If a large dose of these medications is taken or if you are particularly sensitive to them, your heart rate may increase and palpitations may occur. This may feel uncomfortable but does not damage the heart; however, care should be taken in people with high blood pressure and disturbances of heart rhythm. Care should also be taken in people with glaucoma.

Can my lungs get used to my inhalers, and will they become less effective if I take them regularly?

Your inhalers are likely to be of two different types: a preventer and a reliever. You are meant to take your preventer inhaler regularly, and it won't work unless you do. There is no chance that your body will get used to this treatment – in fact, rather than needing to take more as time goes by, you may well find that you can take less because your asthma will come under better control. Nor can you become addicted to these inhalers, although you will probably need to continue to use them for the foreseeable future as at the moment we have no cure for asthma.

Your reliever inhaler should only be taken when you need it, which is when you actually have symptoms or before exercise. If you take it in this way, it will continue to be effective. If you find that you are needing to use more than three to four doses a week of your reliever inhaler, this is a sign that you are probably not getting enough of your preventer inhaler and that your inhaler technique needs checking or the dose needs to be adjusted. In either case, you should consult your GP.

If you have an acute attack of asthma and find that your reliever inhaler is not having any effect, this is a danger signal telling you that the attack is a severe one and that you should seek immediate medical help.

Which should I use first, my reliever or my preventer inhaler?

You will not often need to take both of these inhalers at the same time, because you should take your reliever inhaler only when you actually need to, which is when you have symptoms. Current thinking suggests that it may actually be harmful to use your reliever inhaler when you have no symptoms.

If you do need to take both inhalers at the same time, it makes sense to use your reliever medication first, as it will open up your airways and let your preventer medication get deeper down into your lungs.

How do asthma treatments for young children or infants differ from those for adults?

Most of the treatments used for adults are also effective in children, and you will find that many children are on just the same medications as older people, often in the same doses and using the same types of inhalers. However, there are certain medications that seem to work better in children than in adults, and also some that are not often used.

In children under one year of age, the commonly prescribed reliever salbutamol (Ventolin and Airomir) may not be very effective, so a different type of bronchodilator drug called ipratropium (Atrovent) is often preferred. Sometimes it is necessary for people with asthma to take a corticosteroid medication by mouth; for example, prednisolone, a powerful drug that fights inflammation and allows the airway walls to recover. (These corticosteroid drugs are not the same as the steroids misused by some athletes: those are *anabolic* steroids.) If given in short courses of 3–7 days, corticosteroids are not harmful, but doctors try to avoid using them over long periods in childhood because they can have harmful side effects on growth and on bone strength. You will find more information about all these types of drugs later in this chapter.

The major challenge in treating very young children with asthma is not so much the choice of medication but how to deliver it efficiently to their lungs. We now have a range of spacer devices designed especially for use in babies and very young children, and with the help of one of these it is possible to use a metered dose inhaler (shown in Figure 3) to give asthma treatments to a child of any age. Children old enough to have developed sufficient co-ordination to use an inhaler without a spacer have the same choice of devices as adults (the range of inhalers available was discussed earlier in this section).

My asthma can be very variable, and my doctor often asks me to increase or decrease the number of puffs of my preventer inhaler. He's done this so often that I feel I know as well, if not better, than he does, how much I need. Can I adjust the dose of medication myself?

You are right: the person with asthma is often the one who best knows how good or bad the asthma is at any particular time. However, it is not a good idea to make all the changes to your treatment yourself. If you did, your doctor would never know what dose you were taking or how you were feeling, and there is always the chance that you might get it wrong and take either too much or – more dangerously – too little of your treatment.

A very good and effective compromise would be to agree on a plan of self-management with your doctor: an asthma action plan. Most of these plans are based on your peak flow measurements (explained in the previous section, 'Diagnosis and assessment') as well as your symptoms, because many people with asthma find it difficult to judge how bad their asthma is. Your doctor or asthma nurse will agree with you what you could do if your asthma worsens. Usually you would be asked to alter your medication, depending on your symptoms or on how your peak flow compares with your normal levels. The action you then take would depend on your individual circumstances.

Everyone with asthma should have an asthma action plan. I suggest that you discuss this with your doctor, and ask him or her to write a self-management plan for you which you can use to take more responsibility for your treatment.

My 9-year-old son has been diagnosed as having asthma, and I am worried about both of the inhalers our doctor has put him on. Are the side effects of asthma treatments dangerous?

Before we start thinking about the side effects of drug treatments for asthma, it is important to remember that asthma itself can be dangerous. In children, poorly controlled asthma can cause chest deformities, poor growth, and a deterioration in academic performance because of lost sleep and time lost from school. Your child's asthma can lead to a decrease in the quality of life for the whole family. In adults, asthma can be a life-threatening condition, although it is relatively rare for anyone to die from it. It is therefore important to view the side effects of asthma treatment with this perspective in mind.

Side effects – if any – will depend upon which treatments your son is taking.

Any side effects from his reliever medications will be temporary, lasting for a maximum of four hours after he takes the drug. There are two main types of reliever, and they have different side effects.

The first group, which includes salbutamol (Airomir, Asmasal, Salamol, Ventodisk, Ventolin) and terbutaline (Bricanyl), can cause a fine trembling, particularly noticeable in the hands. Sleep can be disturbed, especially in children. If a large dose of these medications is taken or if a child is particularly sensitive to them, the heart rate may increase and palpitations may occur. This may feel uncomfortable but doesn't damage the heart.

The second group, which includes ipratropium (Atrovent, Respontin) can cause a dry mouth and blurred vision. Occasionally, difficulty in passing urine and constipation can occur.

There is more concern these days about the side effects of the preventer medications. If your son is taking sodium cromoglicate (Intal) you need not worry, as this drug has no known side effects. If he has been prescribed an inhaled steroid such as beclometasone (AeroBec, Asmabec, Beclazone, Becodisk, Becotide, Qvar) or budesonide (Pulmicort), you need not be concerned, provided that he is taking a low dose. (Discuss the dose with your doctor, but, as a general rule, a low dose is regarded as up to 400 micrograms a day.) At these doses, the two most common side effects are hoarseness, and oral thrush, a fungal infection that may show up as a red rash with white spots in the mouth and on the back of the throat. Both of these side effects can be prevented by using a spacer device (examples are shown in

Figures 6, 7 and 8), which will reduce the amount of medication deposited in the mouth, and by brushing the teeth and rinsing the mouth after taking the inhaler.

At higher doses, there are other possible side effects, but these are unusual. Inhaled steroids may cause a child's growth to slow down temporarily; if this happens, the child will experience catch-up growth later, meaning that the child usually achieves normal adult height. Any child using more than 800 micrograms a day of an inhaled steroid should be under the care of a specialist.

In adults taking very high doses of inhaled steroids over a number of years, there may be a risk of thinning of the bones (osteoporosis). This risk is much higher if oral steroid tablets such as prednisolone are taken for prolonged periods (months or years). Short courses of prednisolone tablets (i.e. for less than two weeks) taken up to four times a year are not thought to cause significant side effects. If your son has to take steroid tablets regularly and you are concerned about their side effects, talk it over with your doctor. Whatever you do, **do not stop treatment with steroid tablets suddenly**: this can be very dangerous.

Listed together like this, the side effects sound rather alarming, but all these risks must be balanced against the risks of uncontrolled asthma. Drugs such as beclometasone (e.g. Becotide) have been in use for over 30 years, and have an extremely good track record for safety. People who have been using inhaled steroid medications over a long period of time during their childhood are no shorter than their friends who do not have asthma, and are probably considerably taller than they would have been had their asthma remained untreated.

The safest course of action for your son is to take adequate treatment with effective preventer medications, preferably by the inhaled route, with the aim of gaining control of his asthma, and then to reduce his preventer treatment to the lowest dose that keeps his asthma well controlled. He should then use his reliever inhaler only when he has symptoms.

I have trouble remembering to take the morning dose of my brown inhaler, as I am always so rushed trying to get out of the house. Can I take it once a day at night?

If your brown inhaler contains beclometasone, you really do need to take it twice a day. The effect of each dose lasts only around 12 hours, so one dose a day would not be anywhere near as effective as two. If you are taking budesonide (Pulmicort), this can be reduced to a once a day dosage if your asthma is under really good control. You should take the same total daily dose, and the single dose should be taken at night.

There are two newer inhaled steroids that are longer acting than the others. They are ciclesonide (Alvesco), which is taken once a day, and mometasone (Asmanex), which can be taken once (at night) or twice a day. Ciclesonide and mometasone are only for use in adults.

Will I develop bigger muscles if I take inhaled steroids?

No, you won't. The steroids you are thinking of, which are abused by some athletes, are anabolic steroids; the ones used in asthma medications are a different type, called corticosteroids. Also, using the inhaled route for an asthma drug allows it to be taken in tiny doses, because it goes straight to the part of the body where it is needed. As you can see from the previous answer, there are relatively few side effects from inhaled corticosteroids.

If you take part in competitive sport, you will still be allowed to use both your reliever and your preventer asthma inhalers, but you will have to apply for a Therapeutic Use Exemption to cover the medications you use. You would not be allowed to compete if you were taking steroids by mouth, and you should be aware that several over-the-counter preparations contain banned substances.

I have just discovered that I am pregnant, and I am worried that my asthma treatment could be harmful to my baby. Should I stop my inhalers?

I can understand your concern but there is no need for you to stop your inhalers. Even if you are using a steroid preventer inhaler, this will not pose any threat to your baby's well-being (the side effects of steroid inhalers were discussed in the answer to an earlier question). All inhaled asthma medications can be taken safely in pregnancy. As a rule, it is best to avoid all medications taken by mouth in the first three months of your pregnancy, although if you are taking a leukotriene antagonist (montelukast, zafirlukast), you can continue.

What could be potentially harmful to your baby is what might happen if you stopped taking your treatment: your asthma could get out of control and you could have acute asthma attacks. In these attacks, the amount of oxygen in the blood going to your baby can drop to harmful levels, so it is important to prevent any worsening of your asthma. My advice is that you continue using your inhalers, adjusting them as necessary under your GP's supervision so that your asthma is kept under the best possible control.

I have heard that some asthma inhalers still contain CFCs which harm the environment. Is this true and, if so, what can I do about it other than to stop using my inhalers?

CFCs (chlorofluorocarbons) used to be used as the propellant gas in all metered dose inhalers, but when it was realised that CFCs harm the atmosphere's ozone layer, the government directed pharmaceutical manufacturers to find alternatives. They have been addressing this problem very actively, and most inhalers are now CFC-free, using instead hydrofluoroalkane (HFA). All salbutamol, Flixotide (fluticasone) and Alvesco (ciclesonide) metered dose inhalers, and of course all dry powder devices (which don't use a propellant), are CFC-free. At present, there are only two makes of beclometasone inhaler that are CFC-free: Clenil and Qvar. If you use Qvar, make sure your doctor always prescribes it by name, as the dose of Qvar is half that of CFC-containing inhalers.

The use of HFA instead of CFC should not alter the effectiveness of your treatments. However, when you are switched over, you will find that they feel and taste different from your old inhalers.

My friend, who lives in France, is receiving desensitisation treatment for her asthma. My GP won't perform this treatment for me. Why not?

Doctors have a number of concerns about desensitisation treatment (also called immunotherapy), the most important of which is safety. Sometimes people undergoing this treatment can suffer a severe, even life-threatening, allergic reaction. Because of this, the treatment should be given only in specialist centres that have experience both of administering it and of treating any untoward reactions.

We also have concerns about the effectiveness of this type of treatment. There is little evidence that allergen desensitisation has much of a beneficial effect on asthma, as asthma is not usually triggered by just one allergen but by a large number of different factors. Allergen desensitisation needs to be a life-long treatment, so in view of this and its other drawbacks, it is not a form of therapy that we recommend for asthma, although it is still used in severe allergic reactions and anaphylaxis, and occasionally in hay fever.

There is more information about desensitisation in the section 'Allergy explained' in Chapter 1, and on its use in anaphylaxis in the section 'Living with anaphylaxis' in Chapter 6.

My husband, who has asthma, is very overweight. Would his asthma get better if he lost weight?

Almost certainly. His lungs and heart are currently having to work much harder than they ought to supply his body with oxygen, so, even without asthma symptoms, he is already at a disadvantage. If he lost weight, not only might he feel fitter and healthier but his asthma might improve as well.

I have had asthma since I was a child, but it seems to be getting worse now I am in my thirties. I have been admitted to hospital for acute attacks recently. Are there any new treatments that might help me stay out of hospital?

This rather depends on the type of your asthma. Omalizumab (Xolair) is a new treatment, licensed in the UK in 2005, which can be used to treat people with severe allergic asthma who have a year-round allergy to a specific allergen, demonstrated by skin-prick testing (see Appendix 1). In these patients, the allergy antibody IgE plays a major part in the disease process. Omalizumab is a 'monoclonal' antibody that binds to one particular form of IgE to reduce the inflammatory response seen in severe allergic asthma. It has also been shown to reduce the amount of histamine released by approximately 90%.

Omalizumab has to be given by injection, with doses every two to four weeks. It can only be given to adults and children over the age of 12, under the close supervision of an asthma specialist.

ASTHMA AND ALLERGY

Is all asthma allergic?

Doctors used to describe asthma as being either *extrinsic*, meaning that it was triggered by external factors such as allergens, or *intrinsic*, meaning that it was not associated with allergy. It is now clear that things are not that simple and that there is a great deal of overlap. Most people with asthma are vulnerable to external triggers, but to a varying degree, depending on the individual. As a general rule, the younger you were when you developed your asthma, the more closely it will be linked to allergy. People who develop asthma at a later age seem to have more persistent symptoms that are not so clearly linked to triggers such as allergens, upper respiratory tract infections (colds) or atmospheric conditions.

I was tested recently with skin-prick tests and these showed that I have several allergies as well as asthma. Are there treatments I can use to help these allergies?

When you know that you are allergic to something, it is common sense to try to reduce your exposure to it, as it is likely to be making your asthma worse. There are some suggestions for ways of avoiding allergens in Chapter 9.

Unfortunately, there are some allergens, particularly pollen, that cannot be avoided completely. In this case an antihistamine medication may be a useful addition to your normal asthma treatment. It would be better for your GP to prescribe an antihistamine for you, rather than your buying them over the counter from the chemist, as that way your doctor can be sure that you benefit from it and also prescribe one that is safe in combination with your other medications.

Antihistamines work by blocking the effects of histamine, the substance that is produced when an allergic reaction takes place (there is more information about this in the section 'Allergy explained' in Chapter 1). They are usually taken by mouth, and are available in both liquid and tablet form. The newer preparations cause less drowsiness than the old ones, and some only need to be taken once a day, which makes it easier to remember to take them.

My daughter has just been diagnosed as having asthma. We have a cat, which we regard as a member of the family. Do I really have to get rid of him?

Ideally, no child with asthma should live in a home where there are dogs, cats or other furry animals. However, I do understand your dilemma, as pets are often much loved family members that their owners would be reluctant to lose. If your daughter's asthma is mild

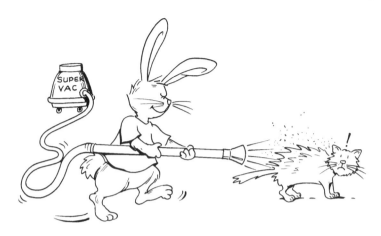

and is well controlled on the treatment prescribed by your doctor, there is no need to do anything about your cat. If her asthma is difficult to control (that means having to use her reliever inhaler more than three times a week), and particularly if contact with the cat seems to make things worse, you need to take measures to reduce her exposure to the allergen produced by the cat. Your doctor should be able to advise you just how serious your daughter's asthma is, and how important a part an allergy to your cat might be playing. He might want to perform some skin-prick tests to see if she is allergic to cats. He might also ask you to think whether her symptoms are fewer when she is away from home in a cat-free environment.

If the cat is a problem, the most effective solution would be to find a new home for him, but be warned: it can take at least six months of careful cleaning and vacuuming to remove all traces of cat hair and dander (a combination of the saliva that cats use for grooming and the scales from their hair or fur). If you want to keep the cat, there are other things you can try. It has been suggested that washing the cat once a week reduces the amount of allergen the cat spreads, but this is easier said than done! Trying to confine the cat to one area of the home and to keep it away from your daughter is probably a waste of time, as the cat allergen is very potent and even the small amount that is spread on the bottoms of people's shoes can be enough to be troublesome to someone with asthma. If your daughter is allergic to the cat and you want to buy some time while you make your decision about rehoming it, your daughter's symptoms may improve if she takes an antihistamine medication regularly.

> *I have asthma that is not too bad in the winter, but it can be much worse in spring and summer when I have trouble with hay fever. Why does my hay fever make my asthma worse?*

There are two main reasons why this happens. Firstly, your lungs may be affected by the same allergens as your nose, which would make it easy to understand why both problems get worse at the same time. Secondly, even if your lungs are not vulnerable to these allergens, any allergic reaction going on in your upper airway can affect your lower airway. Your nose is the top part of a continuous system that reaches down to the very bases (bottoms) of your lungs: if the upper part of this tube is inflamed, the inflammation can spread downwards into the lungs.

It is important to ensure that your hay fever is treated as successfully as possible – not just to relieve the symptoms in your nose but also for the sake of your asthma. This might mean using both an anti-inflammatory nasal spray and an antihistamine preparation taken by mouth. Hay fever is discussed in detail in Chapter 4, and you will find more information about these treatments there.

> *I am sure that certain foods make my asthma worse but my doctor says that food allergies are not a cause of asthma. Can food allergies cause asthma?*

Food allergies certainly exist (they are discussed in Chapter 5) but it is relatively unusual for them to be responsible for triggering asthma. They are only an important trigger in a few people, and these people usually have a strong tendency to allergies as well, and often have a particular allergic skin problem called urticaria (discussed in the section 'Skin allergies explained' in Chapter 3). The most likely foods to cause this type of problem are peanut (the ground nut, not a true nut), cow's milk, true nuts, seafood and shellfish. It is possible to test you for allergies to these foods, and you should discuss this with your doctor and ask to be referred to a specialist, especially if you think that foods are triggering severe attacks of asthma.

If you do discover that food allergy is responsible for some of your symptoms, it is unlikely this is the only trigger for your asthma. Even if you managed to avoid completely any foods to which you have positive skin tests, you would probably still need to continue using your regular asthma medication. If you prove not to be allergic to any foods but certain things in your diet seem to make your symptoms worse, it may be that food additives are responsible – see the next question.

What about food additives – are they a cause of asthma?

Food additives are blamed for a large number of medical conditions but in reality they cause relatively few. Two of the food additives that are known to bring on attacks of asthma are:

- tartrazine (E number 102), a yellow colouring found in many sweets and soft drinks;

- sodium metabisulphate, an antioxidant used to stop food going rancid; it is found in canned and dried foods, soft drinks and wine, and in packet soup, sauces and gravy mixes.

These additives are clearly marked on food labels in the UK, and it would be advisable for anyone with asthma to avoid them.

There are a lot of allergy problems in my family. Will breast-feeding my baby make her less likely to develop asthma? How long should I continue?

Bottle-fed babies are more likely to develop allergic conditions – including asthma – when compared with babies who are breast-fed. Partially breast-feeding (a mixture of breast and bottle milk) has some protective effect. I would recommend that you exclusively breast-feed (with breast milk only), provided that you are able to, and that you continue for at least six months if you can. This has been shown to reduce the number of children developing asthma by the age of 4 years.

There is more information on breast-feeding and food allergies in Chapter 5.

I know that I am allergic to the house dust mite and that it affects my asthma. Is it worth me buying an ioniser or a dehumidifier?

There are a large number of devices on the market that are claimed to help people who have asthma. Among them are ionisers and dehumidifiers, both of which have been shown to reduce the amount of house dust mite allergen circulating in the air. Ionisers do this by adding a negative electrical charge to particles in the air, which encourages them to settle. Dehumidifiers work by reducing humidity and making conditions inside the home a less favourable environment for the house dust mite.

Before you buy either of these (often expensive) devices, it is worth looking at the scientific evidence for their effectiveness, because some of the manufacturers' claims are unfounded. These devices can reduce allergen levels, but not to levels that will have an impact on your asthma symptoms, which, after all, is the result you are after. And they might even make things worse; one study used ionisers in asthmatic children's bedrooms and found that their night-time symptoms got worse. I would not recommend that you buy either of these devices.

Other strategies, as outlined in Chapter 9, are much more likely to be effective in reducing your symptoms. If you are thinking of buying any anti-allergy product, I suggest that you contact Asthma UK (contact details in Appendix 2) for more information.

Both my husband and I have asthma, and we are about to move home. Is there any type of home that might be particularly suitable for us?

By choosing your new home carefully you might be able to make a difference to your asthma, but to do this you need to know what the triggers to your symptoms are. You could think about the following issues, which are discussed in more detail in Chapter 9.

- **Traffic pollution** Try to choose a home that is not on a main road and where it is not necessary for you regularly to walk along busy roads, for example to get to the local shops or to the local school. Check local levels of air pollution by contacting the Air Pollution Information Service, run by the Department of Environment, Food and Rural Affairs (DEFRA; see Appendix 2) or Teletext page 156. Ceefax page 417 has five-day air-pollution forecasts for most areas.

- **Moulds and spores** If your asthma is affected by moulds and spores, you should avoid homes with signs of damp, and ones located near rivers or canals.

- **Pollens** If you are allergic to grass and tree pollen, it would be sensible to choose a home that is not surrounded by fields and which does not have a large collection of trees nearby. Pollens can travel long distances in the wind, but if you would like to have the general details of an area's pollen count, send an s.a.e. and a note of the area(s) you would like information about to the Pollen Research Unit (see Appendix 2). During the summer, look out for regional pollen counts in the local media, or on the BBC website, which gets its information from the National Pollen and Aerobiology Research Unit (see Appendix 2 for details).

- **Animals and pets** If you are allergic to furry animals, you should avoid situations where you might find contact with them difficult to avoid. As it can take many months of vigorous cleaning to remove animal hair and allergens from a home, it would be sensible to try to avoid buying a home where pets (particularly cats) have been kept.

- **Ventilation** In order to be energy efficient, modern homes tend to be tightly sealed with poor ventilation. Unfortunately, the less well ventilated the home, the higher the levels of house dust mite inside it, because the house dust mite thrives in warm, humid conditions. It would be wise for you to consider purchasing an older style of home that has features such as fireplaces and air bricks which increase ventilation.

- **Flooring** Fitted carpets increase levels of dust and therefore of the house dust mite. Smooth floor surfaces such as lino, wood flooring or tiles are easier to keep clean and dust free.

- **Heating** Forms of heating that blow the air around (such as ducted hot-air heating) tend to aggravate asthma symptoms because they increase the amount of house dust mite allergen becoming air-borne. The least troublesome form of heating is gas central heating using radiators, but only when the gas boiler is well away from the living area and the bedrooms. You should avoid open gas fires because these produce waste gases that can trigger asthma symptoms.

What general things can I do to improve my asthma control?

Your question highlights an important point: that your asthma will be better controlled if you take your share of the responsibility and keep yourself well. Your doctor can't do it all for you. You could think about the following.

- Take your preventer medications regularly in the way they have been prescribed and according to your asthma action plan. They will not work if you don't take them correctly.

- Never allow your medications to run out. If you stop using your preventer medications, your asthma will almost certainly get worse. And it could be dangerous to be without your reliever inhaler when you need it. Make sure your medications are on the repeat prescription system at your surgery, and order them **before** you run out.

- See your doctor or asthma nurse regularly for review: at least once a year and more frequently for children and people with severe asthma.

- If you can, avoid the triggers that make your asthma worse.

- Stick to your asthma action plan.

- Eat healthily. At least five portions of fresh fruit and vegetables a day is especially important as they contain antioxidants such as vitamins C and E, selenium, flavonoids (found in nuts, red fruit and vegetables) and beta-carotene (found in yellow and orange fruit and vegetables, and dark-green leafy vegetables), all of which have been shown to decrease asthma symptoms in some people. You should try to increase your intake of omega-3, found in oily fish, flaxseeds, pumpkin seeds and walnuts, and to reduce your intake of omega-6 fatty acids (from foods such as meat and egg yolks, and certain cooking oils), as these measures too may improve your symptoms.

- Drink plenty of water and avoid becoming dehydrated.

- Take regular exercise: 30 minutes of fast walking each day is recommended, but you don't have to do it in one go; three 10-minute sessions are just as good.

- Avoid exposure to cigarette smoke, and never smoke yourself.

3 | Skin allergies

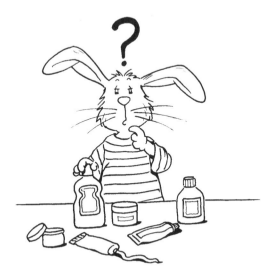

The skin is the largest organ of the body. As it is the part of us that is in most direct contact with the rest of the world, it is not surprising that it is frequently affected by allergies. For example, between 10% and 15% of children and between 1% and 5% of adults have eczema.

There are several different ways in which allergy may affect the skin, as well as many other skin problems that can sometimes mimic allergic skin diseases. Because of this, it can be very difficult to work out whether your skin problem is due to an allergy and, if so, which allergen is responsible. Most people's skin comes into contact with many different substances as part of their everyday lives. There are, however, a number of tests that a dermatologist (skin specialist) or an allergy specialist can use to identify the culprits. Once you know what these are, you can take action to avoid them in the future. If avoidance is not possible, treatments are available that can help to relieve your symptoms.

SKIN ALLERGIES EXPLAINED

Although there are numerous different types of skin complaint, only four are due to allergy:

- eczema, also called atopic dermatitis;
- allergic contact dermatitis;
- urticaria; and
- angioedema.

These conditions are explained in this section.

A child at my son's school always seems to be itching and scratching because of his eczema. Is eczema catching, and should I keep my son away from this other boy?

There is no need for that, as eczema is not catching or infectious in any way. There are contagious skin infections that cause itching and scratching but eczema is not one of them.

Another name for eczema is *atopic dermatitis*; it is a form of dermatitis that happens in people who are prone to developing allergies because they have an inherited tendency called atopy (atopy is discussed in detail in the section 'Allergy explained' in Chapter 1). 'Dermatitis' is the name given to any inflammatory reaction affecting the skin (the process of inflammation is explained in the section 'Symptoms' in Chapter 1). The word dermatitis comes from the Greek *derma*, meaning 'skin', and *-itis*, meaning 'inflammation'. The inflammation causes swelling in both the superficial (surface) and the deeper layers of the skin, and it can be triggered by contact with a wide variety of substances, some but not all of which are allergens.

Eczema is a chronic (long-lasting) form of skin inflammation that tends to vary in severity over time, getting worse and getting better for no apparent reason. It is largely a childhood condition, usually occurring for the first time in early life, although it can start at any age. The majority of children grow out of their eczema, 60% to 70% being clear by their mid-teens, though it can recur in later life.

In mild cases of eczema, the skin is dry and scaly, but it can be red and weepy if the eczema is severe. It has a tendency to affect particular parts of the body. In infants, it can affect the whole of the body but the nappy area is usually spared. In older children and adults it affects the wrists, the ankles, inside the elbows and behind the knees and ears.

Eczema irritates the skin and makes it extremely itchy, which is why your son's friend keeps wanting to scratch. A vicious cycle can be set up, with the scratching making the eczema more severe, so it itches more and causes more scratching.

You've just said that eczema is a form of dermatitis, so what's the difference between dermatitis and eczema?

It can be confusing, and the confusion arises because of the way in which the word dermatitis is used. Because the term simply means 'inflammation of the skin' it can be correctly applied to a number of skin conditions, of which eczema (*atopic* dermatitis) is one. In practice, the term dermatitis is most often used as a shorthand term for contact dermatitis, and atopic dermatitis is referred to as eczema.

Eczema is a form of dermatitis in the broader sense of the word; that is, it is a type of skin inflammation. It occurs in people who are atopic, which means that they have an inherited tendency to develop allergies. Eczema usually occurs in children born into families with a history of eczema, asthma or hay fever, and is often associated with dry skin.

In early 2006, experts on genetic skin disorders at the University of Dundee discovered a gene that, if it does not work properly, causes dry, scaly skin and predisposes individuals to eczema. This gene produces a protein called filaggrin, which helps to form a protective layer at the surface of the skin that keeps water in and keeps foreign organisms out.

If this protein is absent because you have a malfunctioning version of this gene (called a mutation), the skin cannot form an effective barrier. As a result, the skin dries out too easily and the outer layers of the skin constantly flake off. Foreign substances, including allergens, can easily enter the skin and trigger an allergy. This explains the development of atopic eczema, which usually begins before a child is 2 years old, and often before the age of 6 months. In a young infant it frequently starts on the trunk of the body and on the face, and as the child gets older the backs of the knees and the insides of the elbows become affected. It often improves with age, and in many children it disappears by the time they are 4 years old. However, it may become worse again later on in life, and about a quarter of all children with severe eczema will continue to have it into adult life.

Contact dermatitis can be allergic or non-allergic. Only about 20% of cases are caused by an allergy to a specific allergen. In these cases the problem is called *allergic contact dermatitis*. In the other 80% of cases, the skin inflammation is the result of a chemical acting on the skin as an irritant – this type of contact dermatitis is not linked to atopy or allergy in any way, although the appearance of the inflamed skin may be indistinguishable from allergic contact dermatitis.

Allergic contact dermatitis is most common in adulthood, being unusual in children and in older people, and occurs more often in females than in males. The allergens that most commonly cause allergic contact dermatitis are nickel, formaldehyde, and those found in plants and rubber products (these are all discussed in the section 'Dermatitis' later in this chapter). The parts of the body affected by dermatitis are limited to those that have come into contact with the allergen that has caused it.

Treatments for the two conditions differ. The mainstay of treatment in eczema is the regular use of emollients (skin moisturising and softening creams) with the addition of steroid-containing creams and antibiotics when necessary. In contact dermatitis, whether allergic or irritant, if the substance responsible can be identified and avoided, long-term treatment is unnecessary, although steroid creams and emollients may be needed for a time to clear up the dermatitis.

A colleague at work sometimes has red, sore, swollen hands. When we ask what's wrong, she says that it's just her dermatitis but doesn't explain any further. Could you please tell us what it is?

Contact dermatitis can be acute (sudden) or chronic (long-lasting). If it is acute, the skin is often red, swollen and tender, and may be itchy. In more chronic dermatitis the skin becomes thickened and may be scaly.

Contact dermatitis can be caused by allergic sensitisation after contact between the skin and an allergen, in which case it is called *allergic contact dermatitis*. This most commonly occurs on the hands and forearms, which are the parts of the body most likely to come into contact with potential allergens. It is important to realise that allergic contact dermatitis can occur after contact with a substance that has been handled with no problem over a large number of years, as well as with substances to which the skin has been exposed only recently. We still don't know why the skin can suddenly be affected by something that it has tolerated happily for a long period of time.

Contact dermatitis can also be caused by irritant chemicals, which cause inflammation of the skin by the nature of their chemical properties. This reaction is nothing to do with allergy and can occur in anyone coming into contact with the chemical. Its severity depends on the strength of the chemical and how long it is on the skin. If you work with chemicals – for example, in hairdressing, printing, catering, construction or engineering – your employer has an obligation to protect you from any irritant chemical you might work with, and should organise regular skin checks for all employees. Contact the Health and Safety Executive for more information (contact details in Appendix 2).

I have eczema, but recently I developed a different sort of skin
rash as well, which my doctor told me was called urticaria.
She said it wasn't a skin allergy as such, even though it affected
my skin. What's the difference between skin allergies and
urticaria?

Skin allergies (eczema and allergic contact dermatitis) affect atopic
people, that is people who have an inherited tendency to developing allergies (atopy is discussed in more detail in the section 'Allergy
explained' in Chapter 1). They are triggered by allergens and they
only affect the skin. Once established, they can be long-lasting:
eczema can continue for years.

Urticaria (also known as nettle rash or hives) occurs in both atopic
and non-atopic people, and can be triggered by a wide range of stimuli,
not all of which are allergens. It affects about 20% of the general population at some time in their lives. The causes include the following.

- **Allergic causes**
  - allergens such as bee and wasp stings;
  - foods such as milk, nuts, beans, fish and shellfish;
  - drugs such as penicillin.

- **Non-allergic causes**
  - physical causes such as cold, heat, pressure, water and
    sunlight;
  - some drugs, such as ibuprofen (trade names include Brufen,
    Nurofen, Cuprofen), aspirin, paracetamol, and some drugs
    used in the treatment of arthritis;
  - some food dyes, such as tartrazine (E number 102), and
    some food preservatives such as ascorbic acid, sulphites and
    other antioxidants;
  - virus infections.

In some cases of urticaria, especially when it is recurrent, the
cause cannot be found.

Urticaria affects the most superficial layers of the skin, and appears as multiple itchy lumps or weals that are often red in colour. The rash lasts a relatively short time, usually disappearing within 24–72 hours, and gets better without treatment. It is sometimes part of a more generalised allergic reaction, which can affect other parts of the body including the eyes, nose, lungs and throat.

When the same type of reaction takes place in the deeper layers of the skin, it is called angioedema. This can also be part of a generalised allergic reaction that affects other parts of the body as well. It causes more diffuse (generalised) swellings, which are not itchy but can be painful.

ALLERGIES TO DRUGS

Allergic reactions to drugs are becoming more common, partly because allergy itself affects more people than ever before but also because we take more prescription drugs than in the past. Most of the reactions are relatively mild, but some are severe and approximately 1% are fatal.

Not all drug reactions are due to allergy. There are several different types of adverse reactions to drugs, which include:

- a known side effect of the drug;

- a toxic effect caused by an interaction with another drug being taken at the same time;

- an effect due to an overdose of the drug;

- an anaphylactoid reaction, which is like a severe allergic reaction and caused by the release of histamine but without the production of IgE. Certain drugs can trigger this histamine release;

- an allergic reaction involving the immune system with the production of IgE.

The drugs most commonly causing allergic reactions are:

- antibiotics – including penicillins, sulphonamides, chloramphenicol and cephalosporins;
- some heart drugs – including the ACE inhibitors and amiodarone;
- some anaesthetic drugs;
- some cancer chemotherapy drugs;
- some antiseptics – chlorhexidine, iodine;
- vaccines such as tetanus toxoid and diphtheria vaccine;
- preservatives such as parabens and benzalkonium chloride;
- insulin.

Once you have become sensitised to the drug, any further dose will trigger an immediate allergic reaction, with symptoms occurring in less than an hour. The symptoms usually affect the skin, although a severe form of drug allergy, called the Stevens–Johnson syndrome, can affect the lining of the mouth, the bowel and the eyes. Rarely, allergy to a drug can cause an anaphylactic reaction; for more information on anaphylaxis, see Chapter 6.

Some people are more at risk of developing drug allergies than others. Some of the factors that increase the risk are:

- a previous allergic reaction to a drug;
- a family history of drug allergy;
- having a current infection when you take a drug;
- certain diseases affecting the immune system, including AIDS;
- taking a number of different drugs at the same time;
- taking multiple courses of a drug;
- if the drug is used on the skin;
- if the drug is injected, especially into a vein.

The treatment of drug allergy is first to stop taking the drug and then to treat the symptoms with appropriate anti-allergy drugs. For a mild reaction, your doctor will prescribe antihistamines, adding a short course of steroid tablets for more severe symptoms. You can read about the treatment of anaphylactic reactions in Chapter 6.

If the cause of the reaction is in any doubt, your doctor could arrange for skin-prick testing to be done. This should be performed in hospital by fully trained personnel because there is a small risk of a severe allergic reaction. Although using a radioallergosorbent test (RAST; see Appendix 1) instead would avoid this risk, unfortunately RAST is available to test only a few drugs – penicillin, amoxicillin, sulphonamides and cephalosporins.

To reduce your risk of developing further drug allergies, use medications – and this includes over-the-counter preparations – only when absolutely necessary. Use only drugs that have been prescribed specifically for you, and never use medications that have been prescribed for someone else.

Recently my doctor prescribed a course of antibiotics for a urinary infection I had, and the day after taking the first dose I was covered from head to toe in the most awful itchy rash. My doctor now tells me I am allergic to that antibiotic, and that I must avoid not only that one but a number of others, too, from now on. The trouble is that I am now scared that I will react to all antibiotics and I worry about what will happen if I need to take one in the future. Can I be tested with the other antibiotics to make sure they are safe for me?

Many different types of drugs can cause allergic reactions but you are more likely to develop an allergy to a drug that you take only occasionally rather than to one you take continuously. Drugs that are injected or that are applied directly to the skin are more likely to provoke an allergic reaction than those which are taken by mouth and swallowed. Children and elderly people are less likely to develop drug allergies than adults because the immune system is less active at the extremes of age.

In your case, you know that your allergic reaction was caused by an antibiotic. As many as one in 20 people react to the antibiotic amoxicillin, and trimethoprim can also cause allergic rashes. It is likely that it was one of these two antibiotics that was prescribed for your infection.

Allergic reactions to antibiotics are only rarely dangerous, but the rash, which is a form of urticaria, can be itchy and uncomfortable. You correctly reported your allergic reaction to your GP, who will have made a note of it in your case records. As your reaction was quite unpleasant, your doctor will ensure that you avoid that group of antibiotics in the future. There are a number of different groups or families of antibiotics – for example, the penicillins, which include amoxicillin – and if you are allergic to one member of a group, you should assume that you are allergic to all of that group.

It is very unlikely that you will develop allergies to more than one group of antibiotics, so the ones that you must avoid from now on will all belong to the same family; but your doctor still has plenty to choose from. Try not to worry about treatment in the future, as the antibiotics in the other families should be safe for you to take. As the cause of your rash was so obvious, I would not suggest that you need to have any form of testing..

If you do develop similar symptoms in the future after taking another drug, keep a note of the following:

- when you took the medication;

- when your symptoms began;

- how long the symptoms lasted;

- a description of the symptoms;

- any other medications you took during this time, including over-the-counter medications.

This information will help your doctor assess what has been responsible for the adverse reaction.

I developed a rash about five days after starting a course of antibiotics. My doctor told me that it looked like a reaction to the antibiotic, and to avoid taking that drug in the future. I am not convinced, as the rash came on the day I finished the course of treatment. Could it really have been caused by the drug?

Yes, it could. The rash caused by an allergy to a drug can come on as late as two weeks after starting treatment with it if you have not taken that particular drug before – it can take that long for the initial allergic sensitisation to develop. However, if you had taken that drug in the past, you might have already developed the allergy to it and then the rash would have started within an hour or so of your treatment beginning. Allergies do not happen the first time you are exposed to a particular allergen.

Your doctor thought that the rash looked typical of a drug reaction, and so I think you would be wise to assume that you are allergic to that particular antibiotic and to avoid it from now on. If there is a particular reason why it is important for you to be sure of the diagnosis, your GP could send you for skin-prick testing.

I had to have a special type of X-ray of my kidneys that involves an injection of dye. During the procedure I suddenly felt very hot and itchy and got a lumpy skin rash – it seems I had an allergic reaction to the dye. I was quickly given two drugs, and the symptoms wore off after about an hour. Can you tell me more about what happened, and whether it could happen again?

I'm sorry to hear about your experience – it must have been unpleasant and frightening. When people react to these dyes, more correctly called contrast media, the reaction isn't truly due to allergy but is caused by a massive release of histamine from the cells of the skin and sometimes the lung lining, causing wheezing as well. This is called an *anaphylactoid reaction*, which means *similar to* anaphylaxis. The symptoms are very like those of an allergy but do not result from the production of IgE. As far as you were concerned, though, it must have seemed just like an allergic reaction.

The important differences are to do with what can be done to prevent it from happening again, should you ever need to have another X-ray procedure with contrast medium. You should tell the radiographer (the person who takes the X-rays) that you have reacted to a contrast medium in the past, so that they can use one of the newer preparations that are less likely to cause a problem. As well as this, pre-treatment with two drugs that block the effects of histamine, one a standard antihistamine and the other one of the drugs more usually taken to reduce stomach acid, will markedly reduce or abolish any reaction you might have. If you do have any symptoms, they can be treated with antihistamines and a dose of corticosteroid.

I get eczema but only on my hands. Why is this?

This could be eczema, but it seems more likely (for the reasons explained in the answer to an earlier question) that your problem is due to contact dermatitis. I think your hands are probably coming into contact with something to which they are sensitive, and this is triggering your dermatitis.

You need to think carefully about what might be causing your dermatitis, and then try to avoid contact with it. For example, do you wear rubber gloves? These often contain latex, which can cause an allergic reaction. Do you use any chemicals at work? What about other allergens known to cause dermatitis? (You will find a list of these allergens in the section 'Dermatitis' later in this chapter.)

If you cannot identify what is causing your dermatitis, patch testing using a wide range of substances might come up with the answer. This is discussed in more detail in Appendix 1, and can be organised if your GP refers you to a dermatologist (skin specialist).

My baby has eczema. Does this mean that she is going to develop asthma or hay fever?

Asthma, eczema and hay fever are all linked, in that they are all atopic disorders caused by the same inherited predisposition called atopy (discussed in detail in the section 'Allergy explained' in Chapter 1). However, whether or not you develop asthma and hay fever is not only due to heredity; environmental factors also play a part. This means that, although there is a much higher chance that a baby with eczema will go on to develop another of the atopic disorders, it is not inevitable, and your daughter will not necessarily develop these other conditions. Much research is currently underway to see whether certain interventions such as dietary changes, reduction of indoor allergen levels and the use of certain antihistamine medications in early life can reduce the risk of developing asthma in a baby who already has eczema. Unfortunately, the results will not be available for a long while, because such studies require long-term follow-up.

My baby developed eczema very early on – he was only 2 weeks old – and there is a lot of asthma and hay fever in my family. Does this mean he is less likely to grow out of his eczema?

As your son developed his eczema at such an early age, this probably means that he has a strong atopic tendency (atopy is discussed in detail in the section 'Allergy explained' in Chapter 1). Because of this, he is less likely to grow out of his eczema than a child who developed similar symptoms at a later age. But don't despair: only 1 out of every 4 children with severe eczema still have it by the time they are an adult, so the general outlook is really quite good. The frustrating thing is that there is no way that we can predict whether your son will be one of the lucky ones.

CAUSES OF ECZEMA

My baby son has eczema. Why? What causes it?

The predisposition to having eczema is something you inherit, similar to the way in which asthma is inherited, and, because of this, it is a condition that often runs in families. At least one of the defective genes causing eczema has recently been identified (see the previous section). We now know that a protein called filaggrin is responsible for maintaining the effectiveness of the skin as a barrier. If filaggrin is reduced or absent due to the presence of this faulty gene, the skin becomes thin and flaky. It cannot keep moisture in nor keep allergens out. Exposure to these allergens via the skin results in the development of allergies.

Eczema is related to other atopic disorders, such as asthma and hay fever: they all involve an abnormal over-reaction by the immune system to an allergen, which results in the production of specific IgE allergy antibodies. This is known as atopy (discussed in more detail in the section 'Allergy explained' in Chapter 1). I would not be at all surprised to learn that either you or your baby's father, or perhaps both of you, are atopic.

Having inherited one or more faulty allergy genes from his parents, a number of everyday factors might have increased your son's likelihood of developing eczema. These include the addition of eggs and cow's milk to his diet at an early age (before 6 months), the presence of a pet (especially a cat) in the home, and high levels of house dust mite due to good insulation and central heating. Once eczema becomes established, the skin is particularly vulnerable to a large number of substances, including certain chemicals found in skin creams, some foods, and many washing powders: all of these can lead to flare-ups of the eczema. Eczema is also made worse if the skin is damaged, perhaps by scratching, or because the skin has become too dry. If your son scratches, his skin will become more itchy, and a vicious circle will be built up in which the condition of his skin is continually made worse.

Eczema can vary in severity from very mild to very severe. In mild cases, eczema may be the only allergy-related problem. At the other end of the spectrum, people with severe generalised eczema often have asthma and hay fever as well.

The good news is that the majority of children grow out of their eczema as they get older, and fewer than 1 in 4 will have eczema as an adult.

Is there any way to prevent eczema?

Because eczema tends to develop in infancy, scientists are focusing on researching the effectiveness of making dietary and environmental changes in early life. Food allergens (such as those found in eggs and cow's milk) seem to be more important in the development of eczema than those found in the air (such as the house dust mite and pollens). Some research studies have found that, where allergies run in the family, breast-fed babies are less likely to develop eczema than bottle-fed babies. Because milk and egg proteins eaten by a mother are passed into her breast milk, it may be that a breast-feeding mother should avoid these foods in her own diet to reduce the risk of eczema in her baby even more (although before doing this she should consult her doctor). However, it makes sense to limit the exposure of small babies to all allergens as much as possible, and to protect them from exposure to tobacco smoke, which is the strongest risk factor for the development of allergic disease identified so far.

My child's eczema has suddenly got worse. What could be doing this?

There is a long list of factors that can make existing eczema worse. Examples include exposure to allergens such as the house dust mite, cat and dog fur, and pollens; chemicals such as lanolin, fragrances and detergents; and factors such as low humidity, virus infections and stress. Everyone with eczema is different, and will be affected by different triggers. I suggest that you consider the following and see if any of them applies to your child. The list is not exhaustive but it may help you to track down the specific cause.

- **Diet** Is there anything that your child has just started to eat (or has eaten a lot of) in the few days prior to the flare-up?

- **Chemicals** Have you started using a new washing powder? Have you started using a different skin cream, soap or shampoo? Has your child been using bubble bath? Remember that manufacturers occasionally change the formulation of their products, so a product you have used happily in the past may suddenly become a problem. Be wary of the 'New! Improved!' label.

- **Stress** Stress and anxiety can often make eczema worse.

- **Other allergens** Exposure to the house dust mite can precipitate eczema in some people. House dust mites love beds, soft furnishings and cuddly toys. Has your child changed to a different type of bedding recently? Has he been sleeping away from home? Are there lots of cuddly toys on the bed? Have any other allergens recently been introduced into the home; for example, a new kitten or puppy or other furry animal?

- **Season** Many people's eczema is worse in cold weather.

- **Clothing** Eczema can flare up after wearing woollen clothing, both because wool is scratchy and because it may contain natural lanolin.

My child has severe eczema. I am very keen to try to find out if she is allergic to anything which might be making it worse. Can she be skin-prick tested?

Skin-prick testing might be helpful, as you may discover that your daughter is allergic to things that she could avoid relatively easily (allergen avoidance is discussed in Chapter 9). In particular, if your daughter is allergic to the house dust mite, decreasing the levels of this allergen in her bedroom may lead to a marked improvement in her eczema. We spend between one-third and one-half of our lives in bed, and old mattresses, pillows and duvets can contain extremely high levels of the house dust mite. Special bedding covers that prevent these mites from coming into contact with the skin (discussed in more detail in the section 'House dust mite' in Chapter 9) can lead to a dramatic improvement in eczema. However, this bedding is quite expensive, and I would only recommend its use in people who are definitely allergic to house dust mite *and* whose symptoms are difficult to control.

It is perfectly safe for your daughter to be skin-prick tested, provided that she has a large enough eczema-free area of skin to be used for the testing. You will need to arrange it through your GP. Skin-prick testing is quick (it takes about 15 minutes) and painless, but should always be done by someone who is expert in the procedure because it takes experience to interpret the results correctly. You will find more information about it in Appendix 1.

When my son's asthma is bad, his eczema is often much better, and when his eczema is bad, his asthma is OK. Why is this?

Some people seem to have this seesaw experience with their asthma and eczema, although other people find that both conditions get worse together. Everyone with asthma and eczema has his or her own pattern which, incidentally, doesn't necessarily stay the same – so your son's pattern of symptoms may change as he grows older. At present, no one understands why any of this happens, so the only consolation I can offer you is that, at least for the time being, you know what to expect.

TREATMENT FOR ECZEMA

I thought the most effective treatment for eczema was steroid creams. I was very surprised when my doctor gave me a bath oil and an emollient to use on my daughter's skin, neither of which has any steroid in it. Why is this?

Most children with eczema have dry skin, and in general dry skin tends to be less strong and more itchy than normal skin. If your daughter's skin is fragile, and she scratches it because it is itchy, she will easily damage it and her eczema will become a great deal worse.

The bath oil and the emollient (moisturising and softening cream) your doctor has given you are intended to stop your daughter's skin being so dry. If her skin is not dry, it will be less itchy, and she will be less likely to scratch. If she does scratch, her skin will be less fragile and so less liable to damage.

The emollient should be used liberally all over your daughter's face and body at least twice a day, or as often as necessary. If her skin feels particularly itchy, suggest that she rubs in some emollient rather than scratching. The oil is intended for use in the bath but be careful – it can make the bath slippery. Your daughter should avoid bubble baths and soap, as these both dry the skin and can also be irritating.

Steroid creams have their place in the treatment of eczema (discussed later in this section), but the strength and amount used should be kept to the minimum possible, and your daughter should use them only when her skin is inflamed.

Currently, only 'symptomatic' treatment of eczema is possible, using emollients and steroid creams. Now that the underlying gene defect behind this disorder has been discovered (see the previous section for more details), it will be possible to design new more effective therapies to tackle the root cause of the problem, rather than just treating the symptoms.

My mother says that somebody with eczema should not have baths and should not go swimming. My GP says I should bath my son at least once a day using a bath oil. Who is right?

In some ways both your mother and your GP are right. Bathing with soap or with bubble bath can make eczema worse because these products dry the skin. However, if you use a dispersible bath oil (one that mixes in with the bath water), and use either no soap at all or else a soap substitute such as emulsifying ointment, bathing can be a convenient way of treating the skin. In addition, applying an emollient cream straight after a bath is much more effective because the skin is warm and soft.

Your mother is right in saying that swimming can be bad for people with eczema. The problem is not the swimming but the water in the pool! A number of chemicals such as chlorine are added to the water in swimming pools in order to disinfect it. However, if you are lucky enough to have access to a private swimming pool, there will probably be a much lower concentration of chemicals in the water and swimming there would be less likely to affect your son's skin. Swimming in the sea should also cause fewer problems than swimming in a pool (the salt water can be soothing), provided that you can find a clean beach where the water is not polluted.

Whenever I use a bath oil in the bath, my daughter, who has eczema, complains that the water stings her. Why is this happening?

Using a bath oil is an easy way to ensure that your daughter's skin remains well moisturised. However, some of the bath oils made for use in eczema contain a high percentage of alcohol, and even when diluted in water this can sting. Stop using this bath oil, and ask your GP to change your daughter's prescription to one that does not contain alcohol of any kind, such as Balneum bath oil, Cetraben bath oil, Diprobath, E45 bath oil or wash cream, or Aveeno bath additive and bath oil. Be warned: there are a number of other emollients and bath preparations that contain alcohol, and these might also irritate your daughter's skin. Read carefully the labels of any preparation you use.

Rather surprisingly, there are many other irritants and potential skin sensitisers commonly included in corticosteroid skin creams, emollients and bath oils, including lanolin, parabens, beeswax, fragrances, and preservatives such as benzalkonium chloride. If you find that anything you use seems to be irritating your daughter's skin, stop using it and check the ingredients list. If you are concerned, discuss this with your doctor. There are so many preparations available that you can usually find one which is free from the ingredient you suspect is causing problems.

My pharmacist tells me that the product I use for my eczema comes as both an ointment and a cream. What is the difference, and which is best?

Ointments tend to be greasier than creams, and some people find them easier to apply accurately and sparingly. Others dislike the greasiness of an ointment and prefer a cream, which tends to be absorbed by the skin more quickly. Which you use is a matter of personal preference, and may depend on whether you are using an emollient or a steroid preparation or both (emollients and steroid preparations are discussed elsewhere in this section). For example, you might find that you prefer to use an ointment for your steroid preparation but a cream for your emollient.

When is the best time of day to use the skin cream my doctor has prescribed for my eczema?

This rather depends on how often you use your cream, and whether you are using an emollient or a steroid cream, or both (emollients and steroid preparations are discussed elsewhere in this section). In general, emollients (moisturising and softening creams) should be used at least twice a day every day, whether your skin is bad or not. Most steroid creams should be used twice a day but only when your skin is inflamed. Bath oils and soap substitutes should be used every time you bathe or shower. You will find that emollients are better absorbed by your skin when it is warm; for example, just after your bath or shower. It is usually preferable to use your steroid cream after you have softened your skin with the emollient.

If your skin ever feels particularly itchy, a good remedy is to gently rub in a generous amount of your emollient. This is very much better than scratching.

I have heard a lot of worrying things about steroids. I'm concerned about this as my doctor has given me a steroid cream for my eczema. Are steroid creams safe to use on the skin?

Nearly all medications have side effects, even the ones we take for granted such as aspirin and paracetamol. Steroid medications are no exception to this so, as a general rule, they should be used as sparingly as possible. Your doctor will only have prescribed a steroid cream for you if it is really needed, and then only in the minimum strength and amount necessary to bring about an improvement in your skin. If you use your steroid cream as directed by your doctor – using it only on the affected areas of your skin and only for as long as it takes to clear your eczema – there should be no harmful effects. Some of the milder creams (e.g. 1% hydrocortisone) are now available for you to buy over the counter at your chemist (i.e. without a prescription), which indicates that they are safe enough for occasional use without a doctor's supervision.

The side effects of steroid creams are most commonly seen on the skin itself. If they are used for a long time or in large amounts, the skin can become reddened and thin, and marks like stretch marks can appear. The skin can also become pale, or may seem more hairy. Facial skin is the most vulnerable to these effects, so you should take care to use only the mildest steroid creams (i.e. 0.5% hydrocortisone) on your face; if this doesn't clear things up, you should see your doctor.

If steroid creams are used in very large amounts (particularly if you are using a steroid inhaler or nose spray as well), enough may be absorbed into the blood-stream that there might be an effect on the body's production of its own natural steroid hormones, leading to a deficiency of these hormones. This can cause serious problems, including thinning of the bones (osteoporosis), and an inability to produce the extra burst of natural steroid hormones we need when our bodies are under severe stress such as that caused by accidents or surgery. In children, some reduction of growth can occur, although this is very rare.

In order to minimise the side effects of a steroid cream or ointment, it is important to apply it thinly to all affected areas no more frequently than twice a day, and to use the weakest preparation that is effective.

It is important, though, that you use enough steroid cream to adequately treat your eczema, and you should not reserve the creams only for your worst affected areas. If, however, you find you are needing to use them for more than a few weeks at a time, ask your doctor to review your treatment.

There are new steroid creams available now that have fewer serious side effects because they are not absorbed through the skin into the blood-stream as much as the older types. Two examples are mometasone furoate (Elocon) and fluticasone propionate (Cutivate). If you use only small amounts of steroid cream, there is no need for you to change from your usual brand, as you are at so little risk from side effects. The need for a change will arise only if you are using large amounts of steroids, either because you have very bad eczema and use a lot of your cream or because you have asthma or hay fever as well and also use steroid treatments for that. If this is the case, your GP might want to consider changing your prescription to one of these new creams, and you could discuss this when you next visit the doctor's.

Incidentally, the steroids that are used in treating eczema are not the same as those abused by some athletes – those are anabolic steroids, whereas the ones used for eczema are a different type called corticosteroids. Confusion can arise because both are referred to by the abbreviation 'steroids'.

My doctor says he is concerned about the amount of steroid cream I am having to use because I have eczema affecting most of my body. He has referred me to a skin specialist, who has prescribed a cream called tacrolimus. Is this any safer?

Tacrolimus (Protopic) is a preparation that works by damping down the immune response in the skin. It comes in two strengths. You should use the stronger one until your skin clears up, and then switch to the weaker one to maintain the improvement. Although its long-term safety is still being evaluated, because it is a fairly new treatment, it does seem to be safer than steroid creams. The main side effects are skin rash, irritation and pain. You must be careful to avoid excessive sunlight while you are using it, and alcohol may cause skin flushing.

NICE (the National Institute for Health and Clinical Excellence) recommends that tacrolimus and another similar skin ointment, pimecrolimus, are used in atopic eczema that is not controlled by maximal use of steroid creams and ointments. NICE suggests that, because these are new treatments, they should be used only under the supervision of a skin specialist. Topical pimecrolimus is recommended for moderate eczema in adults, and on the face and neck of children aged 2 to 16 years, and tacrolimus is recommended for moderate to severe eczema in children over 2 years and adults.

Good luck; I hope this works for you.

My eczema is much better when I take prednisolone tablets for my asthma. Why can't I take these all of the time?

Prednisolone is a corticosteroid that is taken in tablet form for acute attacks of asthma. Like you, most people find it very effective in these circumstances, but if you take it over a long period of time (by which I mean months or years) it can cause unwanted side effects.

These include weight gain, thinning of the skin, thinning of the bones (osteoporosis) and other serious problems. None of these problems is common, but all are recognised long-term risks of taking oral steroids. Doctors therefore prescribe these drugs to be taken for as short a period as possible, which means for less than two weeks at a time and ideally not more than four times a year: they are then safe and effective treatments, which can even be life-saving in acute asthma.

Your eczema will almost always get better when you are taking an oral steroid medication such as prednisolone because the drug is carried by your blood-stream to every part of your body, including your skin. However, the possible side effects mean that oral steroids should not generally be prescribed for eczema, as it would be rather like using a sledgehammer to crack a nut! Instead, you should concentrate on avoiding the factors that make your eczema worse, and use plenty of emollient (moisturising and softening cream) regularly to make your skin stronger and more flexible, using steroid creams only on the affected areas. This way you will get the best improvement with the minimum side effects.

Occasionally, skin specialists do prescribe oral steroid medications to reduce the immune system's response in individuals with very severe eczema that does not improve with any other therapy. In these cases, the benefits outweigh the potential risks. There are other drugs which work on the immune system that may be used in very severe eczema, and these include ciclosporin and azathioprine.

Just when my son's eczema seems to be under control he starts scratching and we are back to square one. What can I do?

You may find the following suggestions helpful.

- Try to make sure that your son is not coming into contact with trigger factors that could be making his eczema worse. Perhaps there are certain things that you only allow him to do when his skin is particularly good, such as swimming in a chlorinated pool or horse riding, and it could be that these are undoing all of your good work. At least 80% of people with eczema are allergic to one or more common allergens such as house dust mite or pet dander. Your GP could organise for your son to be skin-prick tested if you are suspicious that allergen exposure might be part of the problem.

- Make sure that you continue to use emollient (moisturising and softening) creams even when your son's skin is trouble-free. Keeping his skin well moisturised will help to protect it from damage.

- Ensure that your son can't damage his skin so much when he scratches. Make sure that his fingernails are kept short and smooth, and that he does not wear irritant clothing such as wool or other scratchy fabrics. If possible, remove the manufacturer's garment labels from his clothes, as these can be very scratchy.

- If necessary, you can help to reduce the itching by the use of antihistamine preparations. It is best to ask your doctor to prescribe these for your son, as many of the antihistamines that can be bought from a chemist's can cause drowsiness, whereas the newer types (some of which are available only on prescription) do not have this sedating effect.

- Avoid using calamine lotion. Although it is a traditional remedy for itchy skin, it is messy and not very effective.

- Ask your doctor about wet wrap dressings. This treatment involves applying a warm, wet, open-weave tubular bandage (such as Tubifast) after applying the emollients and steroid creams, then covering this with a dry Tubifast bandage. Gradual evaporation of water from the wet layer cools the skin, reducing the itch and discomfort, and the bandages prevent scratching from damaging the skin. Also, the steroid is better absorbed into the skin when covered by bandages. Discuss with your GP or the hospital doctor looking after your son whether wet-wrap dressings might be an appropriate treatment for him.

My daughter has very severe eczema. Despite using the skin cream, the bath oil and the steroid cream prescribed by the doctor, it is not getting any better. What else can I do?

Firstly, it is important to check that you are using your daughter's skin treatments correctly. If you are in any doubt about this, check with her doctor or ask to see the practice nurse. Assuming that you are using them correctly, it might be that there is something in one of these creams that irritates your daughter's skin, making her skin worse instead of better. Look at the list below, and if you think any of these problems applies to your daughter's eczema medication, talk to your GP about her prescription.

- Some emollients (moisturising and softening creams) contain lanolin or parabens, and these are chemicals that can irritate some people's skin. It would be sensible to change to an emollient that is free from lanolin and parabens.

- If your daughter has very inflamed and broken skin, the bath oil might actually be causing irritation, as some contain a high concentration of alcohol. You should consider changing to a bath oil that has less alcohol in it, or one that is alcohol-free.

- Steroid creams are available in various strengths, and it may be that the one prescribed for your daughter is too weak. Sometimes changing temporarily to a stronger steroid cream will solve the problem.

There might be other avoidable triggers that are making your daughter's eczema worse. The following list is not comprehensive but it may help you to track down the specific cause.

- If your daughter is allergic to the house dust mite and is in regular contact with this allergen, for example in her bedding, her eczema will not have the chance to get better. Some people find that their eczema improves when they take measures to avoid the house dust mite, either by reducing overall mite levels or by using mattress, duvet and pillow barrier covers that reduce contact between the house dust mite and the skin. It would be sensible to find out whether she does have an allergy to the house dust mite by asking your GP to arrange skin-prick testing before buying anti-allergy bedding covers, as these are expensive. You will find more information about dealing with house dust mites in Chapter 9.

- Similarly, the allergens from animals such as dogs, cats and rabbits can make eczema worse, and it would be sensible to make sure your daughter does not have contact with these animals.

- She may be coming into contact with certain chemicals that make her skin worse; for example, the chlorine in swimming pools, the fragrances in toiletries (e.g. soaps, bubble-baths, and shampoos) and the additives and enzymes in washing powders. I suggest that she avoids bubble-bath completely, uses a soap substitute such as aqueous cream for washing, and tries a non-perfumed mild shampoo. You might consider changing your washing powder to one that is as free as possible from additives such as enzymes.

- Her skin will almost certainly feel more comfortable if she wears natural fibres, particularly cotton. However, woollen clothing may be a problem, both because wool is scratchy and because it may contain natural lanolin.

Some people with severe eczema occasionally get a mild but persistent skin infection. If this is the case, the eczema will not clear properly until the infection is treated. This is best done by taking short courses of a particular oral antibiotic when needed, which your doctor can prescribe.

Remember that stress is a factor that often makes eczema worse. It might be worth looking into whether your daughter is happy at school by having a word with her teachers.

My son's eczema has been really bad recently and our GP has prescribed antibiotics. Why?

When the skin becomes damaged and inflamed, it is much more vulnerable to becoming infected by the germs that live on our skin and which usually cause no harm. The infection is usually mild, and can easily be confused with the inflammation caused by the eczema itself. The commonest germ causing this type of infection is called *Staphylococcus aureus*, and this responds well to treatment with a suitable antibiotic. Your son's eczema is much more likely to clear up once the infection has been treated.

I have heard that evening primrose oil might improve my eczema. Is this true?

Recent research has shown us that people with eczema may not have an adequate natural supply of certain chemicals usually found in the body that prevent inflammation. As a plentiful supply of these chemicals can be found in evening primrose oil, further research has been carried out to see if taking this oil can help people with eczema. The results have been somewhat inconclusive: the oil has to be taken in large amounts, and does not seem to be effective in everyone. However, you may think that it is worth trying it to see if it helps you.

My eczema, which is pretty bad, usually gets better when I go on holiday (I like to go to warm, sunny places.) Because of this, my skin specialist has suggested that I try a treatment called PUVA. I didn't really understand his explanation of this. What is it, and will it work?

PUVA stands for 'psoralen plus ultra-violet A'. If this is how it was described to you I'm not surprised that you didn't understand! PUVA is a treatment in which a plant extract called psoralen is taken by mouth. Two hours later you are asked to lie or sit under a machine rather like a sun lamp, which produces a certain type of light called ultra-violet A. This treatment can be very useful in a number of skin conditions, including eczema and psoriasis, and it may produce a big improvement. However, if it is used over a long period of time it carries all the same risks as over-exposure to the sun's rays; for example, ageing of the skin and skin cancers. Because of this, doctors recommend that it is used only to get eczema under control and not as a long-term treatment.

DIET AND ECZEMA

Can certain foods make my eczema worse?

Approximately 25% of people with severe eczema have a true food allergy to such foods as eggs, milk, wheat, nuts and fish. As well as the immediate symptoms associated with food allergy (such as swelling of the mouth and face, generalised itchiness, wheezing and bowel problems), these people may also describe symptoms occurring as much as 48 hours later, such as continued itching and worsening of eczema.

In children under 5 years old, the most common food allergies are to cow's milk and hen's eggs, and eating foods containing these foods may make the symptoms of eczema worse. It is unlikely that these foodstuffs are the sole cause of their eczema but, for these children, eliminating the food responsible from the diet may result in a dramatic improvement in their condition. In adults, food allergy is not usually a major cause of eczema, and it is unlikely that avoiding particular foods will cure your problems.

Food allergy is discussed in more detail in Chapter 5.

Are there any foodstuffs that should be avoided in the diet of a child with eczema?

Some foods are more likely than others to cause allergies, and these include cow's milk and eggs. However, I would not recommend that you automatically exclude these from your child's diet. They are both good sources of protein, and milk is an important source of calcium, which is essential for bone growth in children. Few milk substitutes contain as much calcium as cow's milk. In addition, relatively few children respond with an improvement in their eczema to these restricted diets, which can be both expensive and difficult to follow. (For more information on food labelling, see Chapter 5, 'Food allergies'.)

A more logical approach would be to find out by skin-prick testing whether your child is allergic to any foodstuffs and then to avoid those. However, this isn't foolproof, because small children's allergies do not always show up on skin-prick testing, although a different type of allergy test, the RAST, may be useful (you will find more information about these tests in Appendix 1). In addition, it may be impossible to identify problem foods if there is a 48-hour gap between the food being eaten and the eczema worsening.

I suggest that you decide, with the help of your doctor, whether your child's eczema is being adequately controlled by the use of skin creams and bath oils. If it's not, your doctor will be guided by the results of skin-prick tests and RAST (explained in Appendix 1) whether it is worthwhile considering excluding one or more foods from your child's diet, as explained in the section 'Food allergens' in Chapter 9. You will need the advice of a dietitian if you decide to go along this route.

My 1-year-old daughter has eczema, and my health visitor has told me to start her on a diet free from cow's milk. I am not particularly keen on this, as I feel that milk is an important part of her diet. Can such a diet help, and is it safe?

You are right, milk is an important part of a young child's diet. I suggest that, before you embark on this diet (which can be quite difficult to keep to), you find out whether your daughter is truly allergic to cow's milk.

If I were your child's doctor, I would ask you for the history of her problems, I would examine her, and I would then suggest skin-prick testing to various food products. I might also send off a blood sample for a RAST to cow's milk, which is a specific test for this allergy. All these tests are explained fully in Appendix 1.

I would suggest a diet free from cow's milk only if we found good evidence that your child was allergic to it. If this were the case, I would then suggest that you consulted a dietitian, both to learn which foodstuffs you would need to avoid (it is not always obvious which foods contain cow's milk) and to ensure that your daughter ate a diet that was adequate in calcium, protein and calories.

I have tried to help my child's eczema by excluding foods from his diet that I think might be making him worse, but his eczema is as bad as ever. He is now on a very limited diet but I am frightened of reintroducing all of these foods in case he gets even worse. What should I do?

This is quite a common problem. You have tried your best to improve your son's eczema, but unfortunately your methods did not work. As you have seen no real improvement after excluding all these foods, it is unlikely that you will make him worse by reintroducing them. And as you will see from the earlier sections in this chapter, it is likely that there are many other factors apart from foodstuffs that are responsible for your son's eczema.

I suggest that you reintroduce the excluded foods one at a time, starting with the most nutritionally important foods such as cow's milk and other forms of protein (although, for the time being, avoid egg). If you add one new food to your son's diet every three days it will give you sufficient time to see whether any one of the foods causes a problem. I also suggest that you consult your GP, as there may be other ways to help your son's eczema that you haven't yet considered.

I am sure that there are certain things that I eat that make my eczema worse but I can't seem to be able to work out which. What can I do?

If you suspect that only a small number of foods cause your problems, you might consider eliminating all of them from your diet for a trial period of approximately two weeks, to see whether there is an improvement. If your eczema does improve, you could then reintroduce them one at a time, with an interval of at least three days between each food, and this way you should be able to spot which one is making your eczema worse. You will need to remember that there will be a time lag of approximately 48 hours between eating a foodstuff and the flare-up of your symptoms. You should also bear in mind that there are a large number of things that can affect your eczema other than foods, and that a flare-up could be due to one of these as opposed to one of the foods you are testing. Please be careful not to exclude too many items from your diet at once, and to ensure that you are at all times eating a nutritionally balanced diet.

An alternative approach would be to consult your GP and to ask if he would consider arranging for you to have diagnostic testing for food allergies such as RAST or skin-prick testing (both explained in detail in Appendix 1). The foods most commonly associated with true allergy are all proteins such as peanut, egg and milk, so it is likely that you would be tested for these foodstuffs first.

If you don't yet have any idea which foodstuffs might be responsible, I suggest that you start to keep a diary detailing everything you eat and how bad your eczema is each day, to see if there is any relationship between any food and your symptoms. This will be easier to do if you do not eat pre-prepared and convenience foods (which contain large numbers of ingredients, not all of which are easy to identify) but stick instead to fresh produce and home cooking. Again, there may be an interval of up to 48 hours between eating a food and seeing a reaction. Take this diary with you when you see your doctor, as it will help you both to decide which foods you might try eliminating from your diet or which might be worth considering for diagnostic testing.

LIVING WITH ECZEMA

My daughter, who has eczema, has developed pale areas of skin on her face and behind her knees. What causes this?

Eczema itself can cause *depigmentation* (loss of the natural colour of the skin) but another cause of this is the use of steroid creams. This depigmentation is particularly noticeable when an area of eczema has just recently cleared, but it should become less marked with time. Make sure that you use as little steroid cream as is needed to keep the eczema under control. You will find more information about the use of these creams in the section 'Treatment for eczema' earlier in this chapter.

I had eczema as a child. Now I only get problems with my skin when I'm abroad on holiday. Do you have any ideas why this might be?

There are several things that might be troubling your skin while you are away on holiday. If you go somewhere warm and sunny, it might be sunlight that is causing your problems.

- *Polymorphic light eruption* is a reaction of the skin to sunlight that takes the form of an itchy red rash or blisters, which occur particularly on the face, chest, hands, arms and legs. To avoid this, you should keep out of the sun as much as possible, and you must use a high factor sunscreen when you are in the sun.

- In some people, exposure to sunlight (especially when the weather is humid) can cause 'prickly heat', in which the skin becomes inflamed and the sweat produced by the sweat glands becomes trapped under the skin's surface. This can be quite a problem for someone with delicate or sensitive skin.

- Urticaria (discussed in the section 'Skin allergies explained' at the beginning of this chapter) can also be triggered by sunlight in some people. A diffuse red rash and itchy weals occur, particularly in areas that are only rarely exposed to the sun. The reaction is rapid, developing within minutes, occurs only on parts of the body that have been exposed, and disappears within an hour.

Other things apart from the sun might be causing your problem. The following list may help you to discover what they are.

- On holiday, you might be using certain creams on your skin that you do not use during the rest of the year; for example, a sunblock, sunscreen or an after-sun preparation. These could contain chemicals that affect your skin.

- Your diet is likely to be different when you are on holiday and it could be that you are eating more of certain foods (such as shellfish or cheese), which could be affecting your skin.

- You could be coming into contact with substances to which you are allergic but which you don't usually encounter at home. Examples include certain plants and flowers, a different type of washing powder, or the starch used on the hotel's sheets.

If you can track down which of these things is the culprit, most of them are quite easy to avoid. Failing this, make sure that you take appropriate treatment for your eczema on holiday with you.

Why does my son's eczema always get better when we go abroad on holiday?

This could be happening because he is no longer in contact with whatever it is at home that makes his eczema worse, or because he is encountering something on holiday that makes it better – or it could be a combination of the two! Earlier sections in this chapter have described the factors that can make eczema worse, including allergens, foods, skin preparations and certain chemicals. The change of environment during your holiday may mean that your son's exposure to one or more of these triggers is reduced. For example, he might be allergic to your family pet, or to the house dust mite, and your holiday accommodation may have lower levels of these allergens. It might simply be that he feels less stressed when he is on holiday. Alternatively, it might be the change in the climate that is helpful: increased humidity and increased amounts of sunlight can both help people with eczema.

Is it true that exposure to the house dust mite can make my eczema worse? If so, how can I avoid it?

It does seem that there are specific allergens which can make eczema worse, and the house dust mite is definitely a culprit. Approximately 75% of people with severe eczema are allergic to this allergen; if you are one of them, your eczema may be dramatically improved by measures to avoid house dust mite. In particular, decreasing the levels of house dust mite in your mattress and bedding and using effective mattress and pillow covers can lead to a significant improvement. This is because, when you are in bed, your skin is in close contact with very high levels of the allergen, which can be particularly troublesome if your skin is inflamed or broken because it can't then act as an effective barrier to the allergen.

The reasons why the house dust mite is such a problem for people with allergies are explained in the section 'Triggers' in Chapter 1, and ways to reduce your contact with it are discussed in Chapter 9.

I have heard that it is dangerous for a child with eczema to be exposed to the cold sore virus. Is this true?

If you have eczema, your skin is more vulnerable to all types of infection, including infection with bacteria or viruses. If the damaged skin of a child with severe eczema becomes infected with the cold sore virus or the chickenpox virus, it can be particularly badly affected so, wherever possible, contact with these viruses should be avoided.

If an infection does occur, a medication that can combat these two viruses now exists. It is called aciclovir (Zovirax) and is very effective in treating this problem. If your child has severe eczema and develops chickenpox or any other rash with water-filled blisters, take him or her straight to your doctor because a course of this antivirus drug will make a big difference to the severity and duration of the infection.

We have a cat. Could this be making my daughter's eczema worse?

Yes, it could. Cats produce a very potent allergen in their saliva, which they then spread over their body as they groom themselves with their tongue. Both direct contact with the cat (by stroking it) and indirect contact (through shed hair and skin particles) are likely to make your child's eczema worse. It takes only a very small amount of the allergen to do this and it is easily spread around the home, so the cat could be responsible even if he lives outside most of the time.

It is unlikely that the cat is the only trigger factor for your daughter's eczema, and only you can decide whether to keep the pet. It might be helpful to ask yourself whether your child's eczema gets better when she and the cat are not in contact; for example, when you are on holiday. Rather than get rid of the cat, you might prefer to find a temporary alternative home for him and then see if there is any change in your daughter's eczema. However, you will need to remember that it may take many months of thorough cleaning and vacuuming to remove all traces of the cat allergen from your home.

DERMATITIS

My doctor has told me that the skin rash on my hands is contact dermatitis. What could be causing this?

If your rash is only on your hands, it is quite likely that it is due to allergic contact dermatitis, and not to eczema (the difference between these conditions was discussed in the section 'Skin allergies explained' at the beginning of this chapter). The appearance of skin affected by dermatitis can resemble that affected by eczema, in that it may be red, inflamed and sore, with open areas or scabs. However, in allergic contact dermatitis, the skin rash appears only on the area of skin that has been in contact with the substance which caused the reaction. It usually appears one to three days after contact with the allergen responsible.

Common allergens known to cause dermatitis include:

- fragrances in soaps and toiletries;

- chemicals such as lanolin and parabens found in creams and ointments;

- metals such as nickel and cobalt found in jewellery, zip fasteners, jean studs and so on;

- chromate in tanned leather, matches and green clothing dyes;

- formaldehyde found in cosmetics, newsprint, fabric softeners and cigarettes;

- plants such as chrysanthemums, *Primula obconica* (a member of the primrose family), ivy and tulip bulbs;

- rubber products, especially boots and gloves, which may contain natural rubber latex, mercaptobenzothiazole and thiurams.

It may now be obvious to you what is causing your allergic contact dermatitis. If not, you could ask your GP to refer you to a dermatologist, as patch testing (explained in detail in Appendix 1) may be useful.

I believe that my dermatitis is caused by a chemical I use in my work as a hairdresser. How can I prove this?

Hairdressers come into contact with a number of chemicals during their work, so it is quite possible that your dermatitis is being caused by one or more of them. If this is the case, your hands should improve a great deal when you are on holiday and away from work, or when you wear plastic or vinyl gloves to handle the chemicals. Avoid latex gloves because they themselves can cause an allergic reaction.

As to identifying which chemical is the culprit, the only sure way of finding out is by patch testing (explained in detail in Appendix 1), which your doctor can organise for you. Special sets of allergens are available for testing people who work in occupations such as hairdressing.

Once the substances causing your dermatitis have been identified, it is important that you are told where they are commonly found and how to avoid them. If you are allergic to one of the chemicals at work, you will need to talk to your employer about how you can avoid coming into contact with it.

I have suddenly developed dermatitis. The only possible cause I can think of is a skin cream, but I have been using it for months with no problem. Is this possible?

One of the puzzling things about allergic contact dermatitis is that a reaction can occur to a substance that you have previously used for a long time without any problems. Why an allergy can suddenly develop like this is something we do not yet understand.

So, it is perfectly possible that you have developed a reaction to your skin cream despite having used it happily for several months. I suggest you stop using it and see if your dermatitis gets better. If it doesn't, another substance is at fault, and you may need the help of a dermatologist (skin specialist) to discover what it is.

What are hypoallergenic cosmetic products? Why are they so expensive?

Every time you put a product containing chemicals onto your skin, you are effectively offering your skin an opportunity to react to it. If you are prone to allergies, you risk developing a reaction to any of the substances contained in that product. Most toiletries and cosmetics contain a wide range of ingredients that can act as allergens. 'Hypo' simply means 'less than' or 'lower in', so hypoallergenic products are lower in potential allergens than the conventional formulations. They are free from the commonest substances known to cause allergic reactions, such as perfumes, colourings and preservatives. This does not mean that they are completely allergen-free, but they are more likely to be tolerated by people with allergies.

Hypoallergenic products can cost more than the equivalent conventional products both because they are made in smaller quantities and because the manufacturer may have to use more expensive ingredients. However, several chain stores are beginning to market their own brands of hypoallergenic products that are priced more competitively, and it would be worth your looking out for these.

Beware 'fragrance-free' products: these are allowed to contain a number of chemicals that mask the smell of the other ingredients. Instead use products described as 'unperfumed', as these have no perfumes or fragrances of any kind added.

I am a vegetarian and I get dermatitis. Are there any hypoallergenic cosmetics that have not been tested on animals?

Various ranges of skin care, make-up and other cosmetic products are now available which claim to be 'animal-compassionate' or 'against animal testing'. Only you can decide whether any of these ranges meets your ethical criteria, based on the information given in their leaflets and other publicity material.

Very few of these products are also labelled as hypoallergenic. However, most of the companies that produce them are very good at listing on their packaging all the ingredients used, and some invite customers to write to them with any queries about their products. If you know which substances cause your dermatitis, you may be able to use this information to help you choose suitable cosmetics that will not aggravate your skin.

I can't always find the make-up I want in hypoallergenic ranges, so what do you suggest I do?

A recent change in the law may help to give you a wider choice of make-up, as manufacturers are now legally required to list every ingredient of these products. I suggest you read the labels very carefully, and so avoid any cosmetics that contain substances which you know trigger your allergy.

I have pierced ears, and I've noticed that some of my earrings make them very sore and itchy whereas others don't. Why is this?

I suspect that the fastenings of some of your earrings are made from nickel, and that you are allergic to it. You therefore have a form of allergic contact dermatitis called nickel dermatitis. The

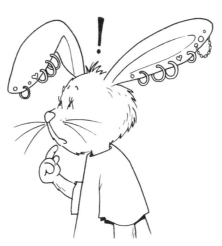

earrings that do not make your ears sore are probably made of gold, silver or stainless steel.

Nickel is commonly found in earrings and other jewellery, and also in clothing fasteners such as buckles, hooks and eyes, zips and jean studs and in spectacle frames, coins and some household utensils. In the UK as many as 1 in every 10 women are allergic to it, and when they come into contact with products containing nickel, they develop inflamed skin within one to three days. This reaction is localised to the area in contact with the nickel, and can be very angry and sore.

I suggest that when you buy earrings in future you check very carefully to see what they are made from, and buy them only if you are sure that they do not contain nickel.

In 2005, new guidelines were introduced offering advice to manufacturers and retailers on how to reduce the incidence of nickel allergy. However, none of these guidelines carries any legal authority, although in some countries, for example Scandinavia, it is illegal to sell earrings or other items of jewellery that contain nickel.

Testing has shown me to be allergic to formaldehyde. I have never even heard of this. What is it, and what substances contain formaldehyde?

Formaldehyde is a chemical that is found in many everyday items such as fabric softeners, newspapers, cigarettes, crease-resistant clothing, cosmetics and some preservatives. If your allergy is severe, you may need the help and advice of a dermatologist (skin specialist), and your doctor can arrange a referral.

Please can you tell me what is in sticking plasters that causes me to come out in a red rash?

This could be due to a number of things. Sticking plasters can contain zinc, antiseptics and fragrances, and all use adhesive. Any of these can cause an allergic reaction. Hypoallergenic sticking plasters are now widely available, but if you are affected even by these, you could try using dry gauze and a hypoallergenic adhesive paper tape instead. You can get these from any chemist.

I'm a keen gardener, but I suffer from dermatitis. How can I best look after my skin?

Be careful in your choice of plants. Because a number of plants can cause allergic contact dermatitis, particularly chrysanthemums and various other members of the daisy family, all such plants on sale have to be clearly labelled with a warning that they can cause skin irritation. Look carefully, as this information may be in very small print on the label or seed packet!

Always wear gloves when you are gardening, avoid rubbing your eyes and face, and don't use a strimmer, which can throw sap and fibres into your face.

Finally, use a good-quality emollient both before and after working in the garden to ensure that your skin is well moisturised (hydrated).

I have worked as a nurse for many years, but recently seem to have developed an allergic reaction to rubber gloves. Is it possible to develop an allergy after using the same type of gloves for years? And what treatment is available for my problem?

Yes, it is possible to develop an allergy to something you have used for many years without any problems. We do not know why the body can suddenly develop such an allergy but, once this has happened, the only effective treatment involves avoiding the substance concerned.

The first, allergy to the natural rubber latex molecule causes an immediate allergic reaction, which can affect the skin (urticaria), the eyes (redness and tearing) and the lungs (wheeziness). In some people this can proceed to anaphylaxis, the most severe type of allergic reaction. You can find more information on anaphylaxis in Chapter 6. If you are allergic to natural rubber latex, beware rubber gloves – these are often powdered with corn starch to make them easier to put on. The latex allergen attaches to the starch grains, which can travel in the air for considerable distances. Because of this, you might experience an allergic reaction if you are in the same room as someone using these gloves, even if you don't touch them yourself.

In the second type, allergies occur to the chemicals used to treat the natural rubber latex prior to use in manufacture, such as the mercaptobenzothiazoles and thiurams. These cause a red scaly rash on the exposed areas, delayed for 8 to 48 hours after exposure.

About 15% of all hospital workers have been found to be allergic to latex, and this figure is increasing every year. Also at risk are people with conditions that require them to use medical products made of latex, people exposed to latex because of their job, and individuals who have food allergy to kiwi fruit, banana, avocado and chestnut. The molecules of these foods share enough characteristics with natural latex rubber that, if you are allergic to one, you may react to another. You can read more about this in Chapter 5.

So, what can you do about this problem? First and foremost, you should avoid all products made from latex rubber. As well as medical equipment, the following contain latex:

- erasers
- rubber bands
- balloons
- condoms
- contraceptive cap
- babies' bottle teats and dummies
- hot-water bottles
- sports equipment (e.g. hand grips and gym mats)
- swimming cap and goggles

- washing-up gloves

- carpet backing

- adhesives

- tyres

- underwear elastic

- shoe soles

- calculator/remote control buttons

At work, you could try changing to a different brand of glove made from vinyl or plastic, made specifically for people with allergies to rubber products. In addition, you should treat the affected areas with an appropriate steroid cream until the rash clears. Because this is a workplace allergy, and your employer has an obligation to protect you from harmful substances, it is important that you contact your Occupational Health department for further evaluation and advice.

4 | Hay fever

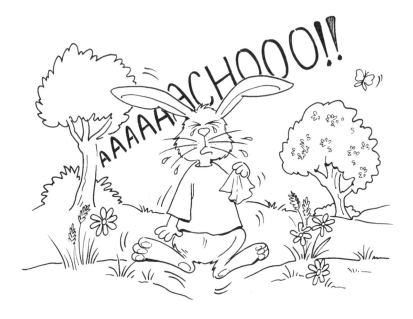

The term 'hay fever' was originally used to describe the symptoms suffered by farm workers during haymaking, but what we now regard as hay fever has nothing to do with either hay or having a fever. It is a very misleading name: fever is rare, and the causes include a large number of allergens other than the grass from which hay is made.

Hay fever is very common, and is thought to affect up to a quarter of the population at some time during each year. Although it is not life-threatening, it causes a great deal of misery. I hope it will be useful for you to learn more about your hay fever, as this should make it possible for you to work out which allergens are causing your problems, to reduce your exposure to the culprits, and to discover how best to manage any remaining symptoms you may have.

HAY FEVER EXPLAINED

What exactly is hay fever?

If you have hay fever, you are allergic to one of the allergens with particles light enough to be carried through the air, known as aero-allergens. The nose and upper airway are designed to filter out any solid particles from the air you breathe, so that they don't go down into the lung. When an aero-allergen is inhaled, it settles on the lining of your nose and throat, which become inflamed (the process of inflammation is explained in the section 'Symptoms' in Chapter 1). The allergen also settles on the moist surface of the eyes, which are similarly affected.

In many people, hay fever is due to an allergy to a specific type of plant pollen, which is only released by the plant at certain times of the year. This causes a seasonal problem, more correctly called *seasonal allergic rhinitis*. The name 'rhinitis' comes from the Greek: *rhinos* means 'nose' and *-itis* means 'inflammation', so rhinitis is inflammation of the lining of the nose.

Sometimes hay fever symptoms can be caused by an allergy to other allergens; for example, the house dust mite or animal dander (the scales from their hair or fur, rather like dandruff in humans). These allergens are not seasonal but occur all year round, causing continual symptoms throughout the four seasons. The correct medical term for this problem is *perennial* (year-round) *allergic rhinitis*. It is, of course, possible for you to be allergic to more than one allergen, and so your symptoms may come and go throughout the year.

There is more information about the allergens that can cause hay fever in the section 'Triggers' later in this chapter.

How do pollens cause hay fever?

Once you have become allergic to a particular pollen, an allergic reaction is triggered the next time that those pollen grains come into contact with the lining of your nose and throat or the membranes covering your eyes. The allergen in the pollen grains stimulates the cells of your immune system, which release histamine and other chemicals, causing the small blood vessels in the affected parts of your body to enlarge. Fluid leaking from these engorged blood vessels causes swelling and irritation, leading to the typical hay fever symptoms of a runny or stuffed-up nose, sneezing and watery eyes.

You asked specifically about pollens, but the same reaction would occur if you had the all-year-round type of hay fever (as explained in the answer to the previous question): only the allergen causing your symptoms would be different. The allergic process involved is the same as that discussed in more detail in the section 'Allergy explained' in Chapter 1, where you will also find more information on histamine and the immune system.

My daughter, who has asthma, is now 9 years old, and has no sign of hay fever. Does this mean that she has escaped it?

Hay fever can start at any time of life, although it is most common between the ages of 8 and 25 years. I am afraid it is therefore still possible that your daughter might develop it. If she does so, it is important that it is treated, because hay fever can make asthma worse.

Is hay fever getting more common?

Yes. Just as with the other allergic disorders, there seems to be an increase in the number of people with hay fever. Increased levels of air pollution may be partly to blame, as damage to the membranes of the eye and nose by these pollutants might make the allergic effect of pollens more potent.

IS IT REALLY HAY FEVER?

Is a runny, itchy nose always due to hay fever?

No, there are a number of other problems which can mimic hay fever. These include:

- the common cold;

- vasomotor rhinitis, a problem of the small blood vessels supplying the nose unrelated to allergy;

- nasal polyps, which are small harmless outgrowths of the lining of the nose, which can cause a blocked or runny nose;

- rhinitis medicamentosa, a problem resulting from the overuse of nasal decongestants (for more information, see the 'Treatment' section later in this chapter).

How can I tell whether I have a cold or whether my hay fever is playing up?

Sometimes this can be very difficult. Usually, however, a cold goes through definite stages. It starts with a feeling of itchiness in the nose and throat, and a general feeling of being poorly; it then moves on to a stage of having a very runny nose; and it finishes with a couple of days when the secretions from the nose become thick and discoloured, and the nose itself rather crusty. A cold generally lasts for three to six days, and then disappears.

In hay fever, the nasal secretions are usually thin and clear and watery, and the symptoms do not pass through these clear-cut stages. However, in severe hay fever, the nasal secretions can be yellow or even green in colour, and you may feel quite unwell, making it hard to tell the difference.

If these symptoms occur at the time you usually get hay fever, it will do no harm to take your hay fever medications.

During the hay fever season, for me June and July, I often get the feeling of having a tight chest, which gets worse with exercise. I had always thought that this was part and parcel of my hay fever, but now my GP has diagnosed asthma. Is she right?

If you think about it, the lining of your nose and throat is continuous with the lining of your windpipe and lungs, forming one uninterrupted system. If there is an allergic process going on in the lining of your nose, it is not surprising that the lining of your lungs could be affected by the same allergen. Inflammation in the lungs causes the symptoms of asthma – hence your feeling of chest tightness, a common symptom of mild asthma.

So the answer to your question is yes, I think your GP is right in diagnosing asthma. It would be worthwhile asking her whether she thinks you might benefit from treatment specifically for this, which, if your symptoms are seasonal, could be taken at the relevant times of year rather than all year round. Effective treatment of your hay fever itself will also reduce the symptoms you get from your chest.

SYMPTOMS

What are the symptoms of hay fever?

Common symptoms of hay fever are:

- sneezing;
- a runny or stuffy nose;
- itching of the eyes, nose and throat;
- itching on the roof of the mouth or the ears;
- a burning sensation in the throat;
- watery, inflamed eyes (conjunctivitis);

- dark circles under the eyes due to blocked sinuses, which may be accompanied by sinus headaches;

- snoring;

- loss of sense of smell.

If you have hay fever, these symptoms often combine to make you feel tired, lethargic and generally under the weather. You may find it is difficult to sleep well, and your enjoyment of many aspects of life, including eating, sporting activities and anything to do with the outdoors, can be affected. You may find that your concentration is impaired, and your performance at school or at work can be affected.

I have never had hay fever, so I find it difficult to understand why my husband gets so irritable when his hay fever is at its worst. What does having hay fever feel like?

The symptoms of hay fever range from a few sneezes right through to a condition that affects the whole body. In severe cases, people with hay fever feel as if they have a bad head cold with a fever, although their body temperature is normal. It sounds as if your husband has fairly bad hay fever.

Imagine a head cold at its worst phase, when your eyes and nose feel intensely irritated and itchy, and your head as if it is about to explode. Your nose runs constantly but at the same time feels stuffy and blocked up. Your nose quickly becomes red and sore, and the constant sneezing is embarrassing. Your sinuses may be blocked, leading to quite severe pain in your face and loss of your sense of smell. On top of all of this you would probably be feeling tired, because you can't sleep, and irritable, which could lead to a degree of depression. This is probably how your husband feels, so it is no wonder he is not at his best during his hay fever season. See if you can help him by encouraging him to go to his GP for a review of his medications. There might be other preparations available that would be more effective.

For me, one of the worst things about my hay fever is the way that my nose runs. Some days it is so bad it is quite embarrassing. Why does this happen?

When the lining of your nose is irritated by pollen grains or other allergens to which it is allergic, it becomes inflamed (tissue inflammation is discussed in more detail in the section 'Symptoms' in Chapter 1). This inflammation causes swelling in the lining of your nose and fluid to leak out of the small blood vessels there. Your nose also produces more mucus. The combination of the leaking fluid and the mucus can make your nose feel stuffy, can make it run (as in your case), or can do both at the same time. Go and see your GP, who should be able to prescribe some treatment for you that will considerably reduce your symptoms. An antihistamine preparation would be best for your particular problem.

Why does my nose itch when my hay fever is bad?

In people who have hay fever, the inflammation of the lining of the nose, which results from contact with pollen, comes from the release of certain chemicals in the body, including histamine (there is more about histamine in the section 'Allergy explained' in Chapter 1). One of the effects of histamine is itchiness. So, in the same way that an insect bite itches, the nose can itch. Histamine production in the nose can also lead to sneezing, and in hay fever this can occur in bouts of up to 20 sneezes.

Some people also find that the roof of their mouth and their ears itch. This is not due to histamine or to pollen landing in the ears, but is the result of irritation of a nerve that supplies both the back of the throat and the ear.

When my hay fever is at its worst, my nose feels completely blocked, but blowing my nose does not seem to make it any better. Why is this?

The blocked feeling in your nose is mainly due to swelling of the tissues rather than to blockage by mucous secretions. Because of this, no amount of blowing can relieve it. In fact, blowing your nose too much or too hard can actually make the problem worse.

A completely blocked nose not only causes local discomfort but can also lead to headaches, disturbed sleep, and a sore throat first thing in the morning (caused by breathing through your mouth during the night). Because of this, I think that you should see your GP, who will be able to suggest some effective treatment – most likely a nasal steroid spray, which will help with this symptom.

Why do I sometimes get pain above my eyebrows and beneath my eyes during the hay fever season?

The bones of your face are not solid, but have hollow spaces in them called sinuses, which are joined to the air passages of the nose by small openings. Air usually passes freely from the nose into the sinuses. However, when the lining of the nose is inflamed (as during a cold or during an attack of hay fever) the openings of the sinuses can become blocked and their drainage system disturbed. Once blocked, the pressure in the sinuses can increase because of the accumulation of secretions. The increase in pressure in these bony cavities can then cause severe pain that can be felt above the eyebrows, either side of the nose, or in the upper teeth.

If this pain persists, see your doctor, who will prescribe an antibiotic to treat any sinus infection present.

My son had a severe nosebleed one day when his hay fever was particularly bad. I found this very alarming, as there seemed to be a huge amount of blood and I did not know what to do. Why did this nosebleed happen and what should I do if one happens again?

One of the functions of the nose is to moisten and to warm the air as it is breathed in so that it does not irritate the lungs. To do this, the lining of the nose is well supplied with blood vessels, which provide both the heat and the moisture. In hay fever, the swelling of the lining of the nose can make it more fragile than normal, and it is more easily damaged. Even quite minor damage to the lining can rupture one of the blood vessels there, which leads to a nosebleed.

The blood loss in a nosebleed always seems to be greater than it really is, so try not to be too alarmed if it happens to your son again. Here is what you should do.

- Keep calm.

- Squeeze your son's nose firmly both sides just below the bony bridge, and maintain firm pressure for at least 5 minutes. Do not be tempted to look earlier to see if the bleeding has stopped.

- While doing this, get him to lean forward slightly to reduce the amount of blood he swallows.

- Mop up any blood escaping from his nostrils gently with a handkerchief or paper tissue.

- Do not let him blow his nose, even if it feels uncomfortably blocked.

- If the bleeding does not settle within 10–15 minutes, or if it keeps recurring, consider seeking medical attention.

If these nosebleeds happen frequently, it would be wise to ask your GP to check your son, to rule out any causes other than his hay fever that might require attention, or to prescribe suitable treatment, which may include the use of an antibiotic ointment until the lining of the nose heals.

Why do I get a sore throat when I have hay fever?

Normally you breathe through your nose, which is designed to moisten and warm the air passing through it. During an episode of hay fever, your nose will generally be blocked, and you will therefore tend to breathe through your mouth. Your mouth is less efficient than your nose in moistening and warming the air, and so your throat can become irritated by the drier air passing through it.

The best way to avoid this is to take adequate treatment for your hay fever, although a short-term answer would be to gargle with a soluble aspirin or paracetamol solution, which will help relieve the soreness. However, parents should remember that aspirin and aspirin-containing preparations should not be used by children under 12 years old.

When my hay fever is at its worst, I have all the symptoms of a cold, including yellowy-green catarrh and a sore throat. When I asked my doctor for antibiotics he would not give them to me. Why is this?

The symptoms you have described could be due to either hay fever or a cold. Antibiotics are not helpful in hay fever unless the sinuses (the hollow spaces in the bones of the face) become infected. Even if your doctor thought that you had a cold, antibiotics would not be the right treatment. Colds are caused by an infection with a virus and viruses do not respond to treatment with antibiotics. As all antibiotics can have side effects, including skin rashes, tummy upsets and diarrhoea, and because excess usage encourages the development of antibiotic-resistant strains of bacteria, your doctor will try to prescribe them only when they are really necessary and likely to have a beneficial effect.

Why, if hay fever affects my nose, do I seem to produce thick catarrh from my chest?

Your nose, throat and windpipe are part of one continuous system. Mucus and watery secretions produced in your nose can drip down the back of your throat and cause you to cough. It may feel as if you are coughing the catarrh up from your lungs, but it is most likely that actually it is being produced from your nose. This can be a very unpleasant feeling, and I suggest that you consult your GP, who can prescribe treatments that will help to reduce this problem.

During the hay fever season I have noticed that, as well as getting a lot of trouble with my nose, my eyes are red and swollen and they water a great deal. They also feel itchy and sore. Can hay fever affect the eyes?

Yes. If you are allergic to pollen, it can cause problems in your nose, your chest and your eyes. The cause of all these problems is exactly the same: an allergen in the pollen causes an allergic reaction, which leads to inflammation.

Most people who have hay fever find that the eyes are affected as well as the nose, because the pollen grains can settle directly onto the surface of the eyes. Inflammation of the most superficial layer of the eye is called conjunctivitis. Allergic conjunctivitis is much more common in younger people, and it disappears by the age of 30 in at least 75% of affected people.

In allergic conjunctivitis the eyes and eyelids can appear swollen, the eyes often look bloodshot, and itching and watering can also occur. The eyes feel gritty and sore, and, in severe cases, bright light feels uncomfortable and there is an increased tendency to blink. Symptoms tend to be worst at the height of the pollen season, which can vary for individual plants.

Medications are available to treat allergies in the eyes in the same way that they are available for nasal allergies. Although bathing the eyes with solutions you can buy from a pharmacy may help, the most effective medications are available only on prescription, so I suggest that you see your doctor.

I wear contact lenses. I occasionally get eye infections, which my optician tells me are because of poor hygiene. However, I am scrupulous about looking after my contact lenses and these infections seem to occur only during the hay fever season. Could they be caused by an allergy?

It is very important that you follow your optician's instructions on handling and cleaning your contact lenses, as eye infections due to poor hygiene can cause serious problems. However, the symptoms of a pollen allergy affecting the eyes can be similar to those of an eye infection. If your symptoms always occur in both eyes simultaneously, I suspect that your problem is caused by an allergy, as it is very unlikely that a pollen allergy would affect only one of your eyes at a time. If only one eye is affected, the most likely cause of your problem is infection.

The most important piece of advice remains the same, whether your problem is infection or allergy – stop wearing your contact lenses at once. If you continue wearing them, you will only make the problem worse. Ask your optician if she can see you while your symptoms are still obvious, as she may be able to tell you the cause of the problem after a careful examination of your eye. If it is an allergy, she could then refer you to your GP for appropriate treatment.

TRIGGERS

What are pollens?

Pollens are small grains produced by plants as an essential part of the reproductive process. The pollen grains, which carry the male DNA, are light enough to be spread to other plants where they pollinate or fertilise them. Although pollen grains are so small as to be invisible to the naked eye, they contain potent allergens that can set off an allergic reaction in people who are already allergic to that type of pollen.

The pollens that cause the most severe allergic reactions are the ones that are carried from plant to plant by the wind. They can be carried in the air for many miles. They are produced in enormous quantities, and because these pollen grains are so light and dry, they are easily inhaled. The pollens from plants that are fertilised by insects tend to be larger and heavier, and are therefore less likely to be found circulating in the air.

I used to live in the country. Last year I moved because of my job and I now live in a city. I thought that this would be good for my hay fever but in fact since I have lived here it has been worse. Why is this?

Many people believe that living in a city should lead to an improvement in their hay fever. Unfortunately, this is not true, for two reasons.

Firstly, pollen grains are very light and can be carried for long distances in the air. The number of pollen grains in the air (known as the *pollen count*) can therefore be just as high in a city as in the country. Most cities contain numerous parks and gardens, which means there are plentiful sources of pollen.

Secondly, although allergy to pollen is the primary cause of hay fever, it now seems that air pollution can also play a role, as air pollutants can irritate the lining of the nose, causing it to become inflamed. Less pollen is then needed to start an attack of hay fever.

The Government has introduced a new strategy to establish national air-quality standards, and will be setting national limits for major air pollutants such as ozone, carbon monoxide, benzene, nitrogen oxides and sulphur dioxide. However, these initiatives are in their infancy, and are unlikely to have a major impact for some time.

How do I know which type of pollen is causing my hay fever?

A number of tests, including skin-prick testing, are available from your doctor which might be able to identify the culprit (they are described in Appendix 1). However, you might be able to pinpoint which pollen is causing your symptoms from the time of year at which they occur. The dates listed below are approximate, as unusual weather conditions can advance or delay pollen seasons:

- The tree pollen season runs from late January to the end of June.

- The grass pollen season runs from April to September, with a peak in June and early July.

- Oil seed rape flowers in May.

- Mould spores are found between May and October.

- Most weed pollens occur between the end of June and the beginning of September.

Knowing which specific type of pollen is causing your problems won't make it easier for you to avoid it, because of the way that pollens are carried in the air. It will, though, allow you to treat your hay fever more effectively. Early treatment is more effective: start two to four weeks *before* your symptoms are due to appear. Once you know the pattern of your symptoms, you may be able to reduce them considerably in years to come by starting your hay fever treatment in good time.

I am allergic to grass pollen. Why, if the grass pollen season lasts for several months, are my symptoms so variable? On some days they are virtually absent whereas on other days I suffer badly.

Your symptoms vary because the amount of pollen in the air varies: they will be worse when the pollen count is high, and better when it is low. The *pollen count* is the number of pollen grains found in a cubic metre of air, and it can be profoundly affected by weather conditions. On hot days with little wind, the count is likely to be high, and it will rise throughout the day to reach a maximum by the late afternoon. A rain shower will have the effect of lowering the pollen count.

Air quality will also affect your symptoms, as high levels of pollutants in the air will exacerbate the effects of any given level of pollen. Your hay fever is probably at its very worst on days when the pollen count is at its highest and the air quality at its lowest.

The National Pollen and Aerobiology Research Unit (NPARU) provides pollen counts and air quality reports daily, relaying information from 33 monitoring stations around Britain. The results are collated into a data bank and used by the unit to provide national forecasts for the media, including TV, radio, Teletext, websites and newspapers. For more information about the NPARU, see Appendix 2.

I am troubled by itching and runniness of my nose and eyes, and these symptoms are similar to those of a friend of mine who suffers from hay fever. However, my symptoms don't seem to occur at any particular season, but happen all year round. Is this really hay fever?

It does sound as if your problems are caused by an allergy of some kind but, as your symptoms are not seasonal, it is unlikely that they are caused by a pollen allergy. The culprit is likely to be one of the allergens present throughout the year. In other words, you probably have *perennial allergic rhinitis* as opposed to *seasonal allergic rhinitis*, as discussed in the section 'Hay fever explained' at the beginning of this chapter.

In the UK the allergens that most commonly cause problems like yours are produced by the house dust mite and cats.

- House dust mites are minute creatures that live in soft furnishings, carpets and bedding, and live off the human skin scales that we all shed all the time. It is the faeces (droppings) of these mites that contain the allergen which can be responsible for triggering symptoms of asthma, eczema and rhinitis. You will find more information about these mites in the section 'Triggers' in Chapter 1.

- The cat allergen is found in the animal's saliva. Because of the way that cats groom themselves, this allergen is spread widely over the cat's fur, and from there it is transferred onto carpets, furnishings, and the hands and clothing of anyone handling the cat. This allergen can be responsible for triggering chest, skin and nose problems in susceptible people.

You need to work out which allergen is causing your problems: although it is most likely to be from cats or the house dust mite, it could be something else entirely. Your GP will be able to help you with this by taking a careful account of your symptoms, by examining you, and perhaps by performing some tests (they are described in Appendix 1). You can then take steps to reduce your exposure to the allergen responsible (see the suggestions in the various sections on allergen avoidance in Chapter 9), which should help to reduce your symptoms. Your GP will also be able to offer you effective treatment for any symptoms that remain.

TREATMENT

There are now so many remedies available for hay fever that I get confused. What is the best medicine for hay fever?

This rather depends on what your symptoms are. If you have sneezing and a runny nose, an antihistamine medication will help, either by mouth or as a nasal spray. If you have a blocked nose, a steroid nasal spray will be more effective. These two different types of medication can be used safely in combination if, for example, you have a blocked but runny nose. Anti-allergy eye drops should be added if you have symptoms affecting your eyes, such as soreness, grittiness and excess tear production. If you take an antihistamine tablet or syrup for nasal symptoms, this will have the added benefit of treating your eye symptoms as well. Several different manufacturers make anti-allergy preparations, so there is a wide range your GP can choose from. If you have very disabling symptoms, these can occasionally justify the use of oral corticosteroids for short periods; for example, for students taking important examinations.

In addition to these medications, allergen avoidance will help. There are many practical ways in which you can avoid exposure to high levels of pollen, and these are described in Chapter 9.

I know that there are plenty of medications that I can get from my doctor and from the chemist to help suppress the symptoms of my hay fever. If I can, though, I would like to use these as little as possible. Do you have any practical suggestions as to how I can try to control my symptoms without the use of drugs?

Firstly, I want to reassure you that all of the drugs available for the treatment of hay fever have been carefully researched and evaluated and, if used according to their instructions, are completely safe. However, I can understand your desire to take as little medication as possible. There are ways in which you can reduce your exposure to the allergens causing your symptoms, and they are described in the various sections on allergen avoidance in Chapter 9. Reduced exposure means fewer symptoms, and fewer symptoms mean that you will need less treatment.

Are there medicines that I can buy from the chemist to treat my hay fever?

Yes, there are several quite effective medications that you can buy from your pharmacist over the counter (without a prescription), and the range available is frequently being added to. However, please don't feel that hay fever is a trivial problem that your doctor would not think worth a consultation. The symptoms of hay fever can have a profound effect upon your quality of life, and your GP will be pleased to help.

The following types of medication can be bought from your pharmacist without prescription, and they are all discussed in more detail elsewhere in this section.

- *Oral antihistamines*, in both tablet and liquid form. There are two main types:
  - those that cause drowsiness, such as chlorphenamine (Piriton) and promethazine (Phenergan). These can be helpful to use at night if you find it difficult to sleep, but be aware that you might still feel sleepy the next day, and if affected, shouldn't drive or operate machinery;
  - newer medicines that cause less or no drowsiness, such as cetirizine (Zirtek Allergy), loratadine (Clarityn Allergy) and acrivastine (Benadryl Allergy Relief).

  Many people prefer to use the newer medicines because these don't affect the ability to get on with daily activities, and many of them have the added bonus that they need to be taken only once a day.

- *Antihistamine nasal sprays*. The only antihistamine that can be used directly in the nose is azelastine. One preparation (Aller-eze nasal spray) can be bought over the counter, and the other (Rhinolast) is available only with a prescription. These can be used to provide rapid relief from sneezing, itching and runny nose, but have no effect on other symptoms such as itchy eyes.

- *Antihistamine eye drops* can be useful if eye symptoms are your biggest problem. They include antazoline and azelastine (Aller-eze eye drops), which you can buy from pharmacies. These provide rapid relief from itchy, red, watery eyes.

- *Nasal corticosteroids*. There are two steroid nasal preparations that can be bought from pharmacies: beclometasone (Beconase hay fever nasal spray) and fluticasone (Flixonase allergy nasal spray). Nasal steroids reduce inflammation in the nasal passages and are better than oral antihistamines at relieving most nasal symptoms, including a blocked nose.

Nasal corticosteroids have to be used regularly to be effective, and can take up to two weeks have an effect. Because of this, they are best started a couple of weeks before you expect your symptoms to begin.

- *Nasal cromoglicate*. Nasal sprays containing sodium cromoglicate (Rynacrom and Vividrin nasal spray) are also used to prevent nasal symptoms. Like nasal corticosteroids, they should be started a couple of weeks before the pollen season begins. They are often less effective than nasal corticosteroids, but may be used in children if there are concerns about the potential side effects of nasal steroids.

- *Cromoglicate eye drops*. Drops containing sodium cromoglicate (Clarityn allergy eye drops, Optrex allergy eye drops) or nedocromil sodium (Rapitil eye drops) should be used regularly, as with nasal cromoglicate products, to prevent the allergic reaction from occurring.

- *Decongestant nasal sprays and nose drops* containing decongestants such as xylometazoline (Otrivine nasal spray, Sudafed nasal spray) can be bought over the counter to treat a blocked nose.

  These can be very effective in the short term, but should not be used on a regular basis because they can lead to thinning and drying of the lining of the nose, and can make your problem worse rather than better. They can also cause 'rebound congestion' when you stop using them.

- *Decongestant tablets* containing drugs such as pseudoephedrine (Sudafed tablets) are not particularly effective, although they do not cause rebound nasal congestion when stopped.

Do consult your pharmacist if you have any questions or concerns about using these medications and, in particular, if you are pregnant or breast-feeding.

My friend and I both have hay fever. She swears by an antihistamine tablet that her doctor has given her. However, whenever I have tried using antihistamines, I have felt really sleepy and rather knocked out. Why is this?

In the past, the antihistamine preparations that were available were effective but had considerable side effects, the main one of which was to make people feel sleepy. Newer preparations are now available that do not have this side effect. I suggest that you arrange to see your GP and ask for one of these newer, 'non-sedating' preparations, which include cetirizine (Zirtek), levocetirizine (Xyzal), loratadine (Clarityn), and desloratadine (Neoclarityn). Some of these preparations are available only on prescription, but it is now possible to buy some of them over the counter from your pharmacist. These newer drugs also have the advantage that they only need to be taken once a day.

If for any reason you continue to use a preparation that makes you feel sleepy, please remember that this can make it dangerous for you to drive or to operate any machinery, and that alcohol will make the sleepiness worse.

I recently went to the chemist's to collect my prescription for erythromycin, the antibiotic that I take for acne, and to buy some more of my antihistamine hay fever tablets – they contain terfenadine. The pharmacist said she couldn't sell me the antihistamines that I've been using up till now, because they have been withdrawn. Apparently the combination of the two drugs was dangerous. Is this really true? They were the only ones that didn't make me sleepy, so what do I do about my antihistamines now?

Sometimes taking two medications at the same time can cause side effects that do not occur if each medication is taken separately. One example of this is when the antihistamine terfenadine (Triludan) is taken by someone who is also taking the antibiotic erythromycin (e.g. Erymax, Erythroped and Erythrocin). In certain people this combination can cause heart-beat irregularities: although this problem is very rare, it is important that no one takes these two drugs together. Your pharmacist was absolutely correct in what she did. To prevent anyone accidentally combining these drugs in the future, terfenadine has been withdrawn.

Your problem about what to do about your antihistamines is easily solved by telling your GP about your hay fever symptoms and asking for a prescription for a non-sedating antihistamine that can be combined safely with the antibiotic you take for your acne. You might want to try fexofenadine (Telfast), a derivative of terfenadine that is safe to take with erythromycin.

I used to use a nasal medication that came as an inhaler. My GP has recently changed my prescription and I have now been given a liquid nasal spray. Why is this?

There are two reasons. Firstly, liquid preparations are distributed much more effectively in the nose, and are therefore better at treating the whole of the nasal lining. Secondly, until recently aerosol inhalers often contained CFCs (chlorofluorocarbons), which are known to be harmful to the atmosphere. All products produced in the European Union must be CFC-free wherever possible. I expect you will find that the new preparation works at least as well as, if not better than, your old one.

When you use your spray, it is important that you use it correctly. Lean forward so that your head is upside down and pump the spray into one nostril. Before you pump it again, briefly hold the spray the right way up so that it can refill. Then treat the other nostril. If you find this position uncomfortable, lie on the bed on your back with your head hanging off the end of the bed, and then use the spray in the way already described. These positions are both shown in Figure 9.

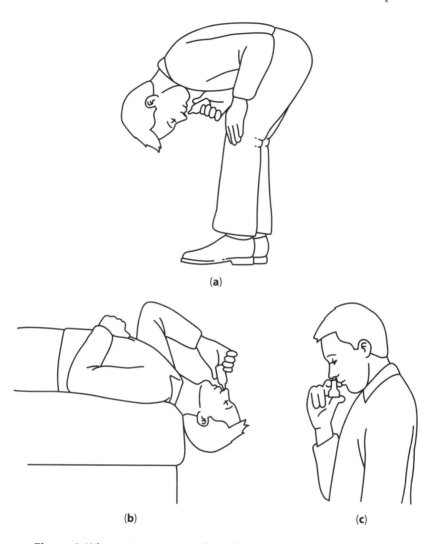

(a)

(b)

(c)

Figure 9 When using an aerosol nasal spray, you can either (**a**) lean forward so that your head is upside down or (**b**) lie on your back on the bed with your head hanging off the end of the bed. For an aqueous nasal spray, you can tilt your head forward slightly (**c**) and squirt the spray up your nose. Remember to blow your nose first!

In the past my hay fever has only affected my nose, but this year my eyes are itchy and sore all the time, and weep continuously. What can I do?

If you are not already using antihistamine tablets (discussed earlier in this section), I suggest that you start taking them. Choose a non-sedating preparation such as those containing cetirizine or loratadine. If antihistamines alone are not effective, you may find that anti-allergy eye drops such as those containing sodium cromoglicate (e.g. Hay-Crom Aqueous, Opticrom Allergy and Vividrin) or a steroid preparation will help. Finally, bathing your eyes with a solution such as Optrex that you can buy from the chemist's will wash away any pollen grains in contact with the eye and may be soothing.

In addition, it would be sensible for you to avoid going outside at times of day when the pollen count is high, and to try wearing glasses or sunglasses while you are outside. You could also try showering and washing your hair when you get home to remove any pollen grains, then changing into clean clothes that have been dried indoors rather than outside where they can become covered in pollen. Dry your bedding indoors too, and keep your bedroom window closed. You will find more suggestions for reducing your exposure to pollen in Chapter 9.

My GP has prescribed eye drops for my hay fever, but he did not explain to me how I should use them. What is the best way of putting eye drops into my eye?

The easiest way is gently to pull your lower eyelid away from your eye and to place the drops into the space between your lower eyelid and your eyeball (as shown in Figure 10). When you blink, which will probably be immediately, the drops will be spread over the whole surface of your eye.

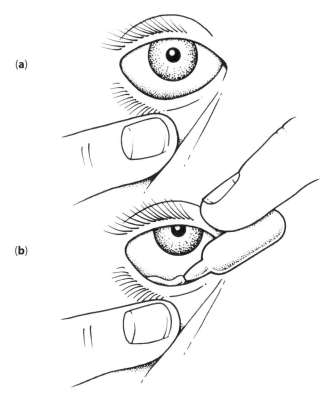

Figure 10 When using eye drops, (**a**) gently pull your lower eyelid away from your eye and (**b**) place the drops into the space between your lower eyelid and your eyeball

None of the medications that my GP gives me for my hay fever is as effective as the decongestant spray that I can buy from my chemist. Why can't I just continue to use this nose spray?

Decongestant nasal sprays have an almost immediate effect and can make your nose feel much clearer. They work by decreasing the blood flow to the lining of the nose which, in the short term, reduces the swelling. However, if these preparations are used over a prolonged period of time (by which I mean for more than a couple of days), they can lead to lasting damage, as the lining of the nose shrinks and dries out (this is called rhinitis medicamentosa). When you stop using these sprays, you will find that your nose becomes even more blocked than before, due to what is called rebound nasal congestion.

Decongestant tablets (which usually contain a combination of an antihistamine and a decongestant) do not cause this problem but, again, they should not be used long-term.

I know that the medications given to you by your doctor do not have an immediate beneficial effect but, if you persevere with them and take them as prescribed, they should relieve your symptoms without causing any damage.

My GP has told me not to use decongestant nose sprays for my hay fever and has instead prescribed me a steroid nasal spray. Surely these can have as many or more side effects than the old spray I was using?

Almost all medications have side effects, even the ones we take for granted such as aspirin and paracetamol. When doctors decide which drugs to prescribe, they have to weigh up the likely benefits against these side effects.

In the case of decongestant nasal sprays, the answer is clear cut. Prolonged use is always damaging to the nose (as explained in the answer to the previous question) and the beneficial effects are not long-lasting.

In the case of steroid sprays, the balance is very much in favour of the beneficial effects. The dose of steroid delivered by these sprays is extremely small, and very unlikely to have any generalised effect on the body. They are given locally onto the part of the body where they are needed, so they can therefore be given in such small doses that side effects are negligible.

Incidentally, the steroids that are used in these nasal sprays and in some anti-allergy eye drops are not the same as those abused by some athletes. Those are anabolic steroids; the ones used for hay fever are a different type called corticosteroids.

Can hay fever treatment interfere with the contraceptive pill?

Whenever you are prescribed a new medication by your doctor, or buy a medication over the counter at the chemist's, it is important that you tell the doctor or pharmacist about any other medications you are taking. So your question is very sensible, but in this case I do not think you have anything to worry about. None of the antihistamine medications or the nasal sprays for hay fever affects the effectiveness of the contraceptive pill.

In the past when my hay fever was particularly bad, my GP used to give me an injection of something called Kenalog. This was very effective. My new GP is very reluctant to give me this. Why?

Kenalog (generic name triamcinolone) is a steroid preparation, given by injection, that has a long duration of action. Steroid preparations can be very effective, but they can also have considerable side effects. In the case of steroid injections these include thinning of the bones (osteoporosis), thinning of the skin, weakening of the muscles and, in children, slower growth. In addition, Kenalog can cause scarring at the site of the injection. If your hay fever can be controlled effectively by using other medications such as steroid nasal sprays (which contain a very much smaller dose than an injection) and antihistamine tablets, this would be much safer for you in the long run.

I read that desensitising injections can be very effective in hay fever. However, my GP says that these are not available now because they are dangerous. Is this true?

Desensitising injections are no longer administered in GPs' surgeries because a few people have suffered serious reactions to them, some of which have been fatal. Because of this, this type of treatment, also called immunotherapy, is carried out in specialist hospital clinics. It is most commonly used for allergic rhinitis caused by pollen allergy and severe allergic reactions to bee and wasp stings. In carefully chosen patients, this can be a very effective form of treatment, and the beneficial effects can last well after the treatment has finished. However, it is time-consuming and the duration of the course of treatment is long – at least two years. You will find more information about it in the section 'Allergy explained' in Chapter 1.

A new type of immunotherapy is now available for the treatment of hay fever. The doses of allergen are given under the tongue (sublingual), which means that injections are not needed. Although this new treatment is not as effective as standard immunotherapy, you might want to try sublingual immunotherapy, or you could use the more conventional therapies such as antihistamine preparations and steroid nasal sprays.

Are there any complementary remedies that are likely to be helpful in my hay fever?

Homeopathic remedies containing eyebright (*Euphrasia officinalis*) or onion may be helpful. In addition, traditional herbal remedies that include garlic are thought to help hay fever and catarrh. Acupuncture has also been successful in both the prevention and the treatment of hay fever symptoms.

I discuss the place of complementary therapies in treating allergies in Chapter 10, where you will find more information on homeopathy, herbal medicine and acupuncture.

LIVING WITH HAY FEVER

I like to go out for a walk each day. Is there a time of day that is least likely to provoke my hay fever?

The best times for you to be outdoors are early in the morning and in the late evening. During the day, the pollens produced by plants and trees are carried up into the atmosphere by warm air currents and therefore the pollen count rises, reaching a peak in the late afternoon and early evening. The air then begins to cool, and the pollen grains fall back down to earth.

You could also go out when it has been raining, as showers clear the air of pollen grains. If there is a rain shower in the afternoon or early evening, the air will remain fairly clear of pollen grains until the following day.

I plan to have an early holiday this year, which will be right in the middle of my hay fever season. Is there anything I can do to avoid a miserable holiday?

If you are planning a holiday in Britain, I suggest that you try a seaside resort. Sea breezes often reduce the pollen count by the coast, especially on the west coast.

If you are planning a trip to Europe, I suggest that you choose a country such as Greece or Turkey, where the vegetation is very different from that in Britain. This would considerably reduce your chances of encountering the type of pollen that causes your hay fever.

If you have enough time and money to travel long distances, a trip to the southern hemisphere would almost certainly ensure you a symptom-free holiday, as instead of spring it would be autumn there.

Wherever you go, make sure that you have sufficient supplies of your hay fever medications so that you can continue to take them throughout your holiday.

I drive a great deal in my job. Can I safely drive when I am using medicines for my hay fever?

You don't say what treatment you are taking for your hay fever, so I can only answer in general terms. Nasal sprays and anti-allergy eye drops will not affect your ability to drive safely. Antihistamine tablets may: some of these medications cause drowsiness, whereas others do not. Most decongestant tablets contain a sedating antihistamine, so those might also make you drowsy. The sedating antihistamines include:

- alimemazine (trimeprazine)
- buclizine
- chlorphenamine (chlorpheniramine)
- cinnarizine
- clemastine
- cyclizine
- cyproheptadine
- hydroxyzine
- ketotifen
- meclozine
- promethazine

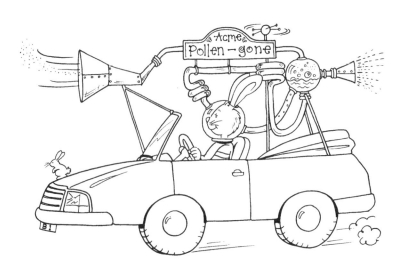

The antihistamines that are thought not to cause sedation include:

- acrivastine
- cetirizine
- desloratadine
- fexofenadine
- levocetirizine
- loratadine
- mizolastine

You should also realise that the symptoms of hay fever can themselves affect your ability to drive safely, so your best option is to take effective medication that does not have a sedative effect.

I suggest that you discuss your current treatment with your GP or pharmacist, remembering to tell them about the amount you have to drive. Most people whose work depends on a clean driving licence are extremely careful not to drink and drive, but it is as important not to drive if adversely affected by prescription drugs. If you decide to try a new hay fever medication at any time in the future, you should have the discussion again.

If you are able to choose what type of car you drive, consider changing to a model that has an integral pollen filter in the ventilation system, to reduce your exposure to the allergens that trigger your hay fever. Unfortunately, these filters have virtually no effect on chemical air pollution (they only remove particles from the air), something to which you are invariably exposed when you drive a great deal and which can make hay fever worse.

I love gardening but I get terrible hay fever! Do you have any tips to help me cope with my hay fever while I am in the garden?

Yes, and you will find them in Chapter 9. I also suggest that you see your GP, who may be able to give you some treatment to control your symptoms.

I am pregnant and my hay fever seems a great deal worse. Why is this?

Pregnancy can have an effect, albeit an unpredictable one, on a number of medical conditions, including hay fever. In some women it gets better, in others it gets a great deal worse. However, your particular problem may have nothing to do with your hay fever. Many pregnant women experience a feeling of nasal obstruction during pregnancy, and this is thought to be due to a general increase in blood circulation, which can cause swelling in the lining of the nose.

I suggest that you consult your GP, who will make sure that you have the best possible treatment for your hay fever and that your medications are safe to continue during pregnancy. Unfortunately, as with many of the effects of pregnancy, it may be that this is something that you will have to put up with until after your baby is born.

Is it true that I shouldn't drink alcohol while I am taking antihistamines?

It is probably safest to limit your alcohol intake or to avoid alcohol altogether when you are taking antihistamine medications. You should be particularly careful about this if you are taking one of the older types (listed a little earlier in this section), as these can be quite sedating in themselves and can interact with alcohol to make you very drowsy indeed. The newer antihistamines – which include cetirizine (Zirtek), desloratadine (Neoclarityn), fexofenadine (Telfast), levocetirizine (Xyzal), loratadine (Clarityn) and mizolastine (Mizollen) – do not usually cause drowsiness, but it is still advisable not to combine them with alcohol.

In the summer I seem to lose my enjoyment of food. Is this because of my antihistamines?

No, I think your hay fever itself will be the cause. The two senses of taste and smell are very closely related: in fact it is often the smell of food rather than its taste that gives it its appeal. You may have noticed that your food does not taste as good as usual when you have a cold and your nose is blocked. In the same way, the smell of your food – and therefore its taste – is lost when your nose is blocked because of the effects of hay fever. It sounds as if your antihistamines are not preventing all of your symptoms, so you might benefit from a steroid nasal spray which can be prescribed for you by your GP.

My daughter seems to have a runny nose all year round. I have noticed that recently she seems to turn the volume on the TV up very loud because she can't hear very well. Could this be due to her allergy too?

Possibly. The nose and the ears are linked by small tubes called the Eustachian (or pharyngotympanic) tubes, which are there to drain the middle ear and to equalise the pressure between the ears and the throat. The Eustachian tubes can become blocked if the nose and throat are inflamed, and an allergy can be responsible for this inflammation. The blockage can cause fluid to collect in the middle ear, a condition called 'glue ear' which can affect the hearing.

As even a minor degree of hearing loss can cause problems with schooling, I suggest you take your daughter to your GP, who can prescribe medications that may help. If the problem continues, your daughter may need to be referred to an ear, nose and throat (ENT) specialist for further treatment.

The skin around my nose and mouth gets very sore sometimes, especially when my nose is very runny. Is there anything I can do to stop this happening?

For immediate first aid, I suggest that you try putting petroleum jelly (e.g. Vaseline) onto the skin of your nose and lips first thing in the morning, and reapply it regularly during the day. To try to prevent this problem, you will need to go and see your GP, and ask whether there are any medications you could use to stop your nose running so much. You don't mention what treatment you currently use, but your hay fever sounds bad enough to warrant the use of both an oral antihistamine and a steroid nasal spray.

5 | Food allergies

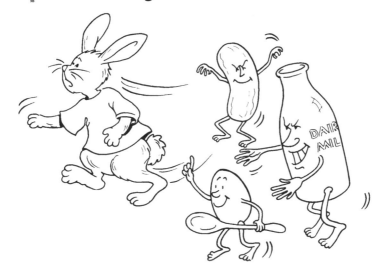

Food allergy affects approximately 2% of the UK population, but as many as 45% of us experience some kind of food-related condition such as intolerance and sensitivity. Explanations of each of these conditions can be found in the next section, 'Food allergies explained'. It's clear that the majority of people who have unpleasant reactions to one or more foods are not in fact allergic to that food. Does this mean that they are imagining their symptoms? Of course not. Their symptoms are real and foodstuffs are, in some way, responsible. Although the treatment of the different conditions may well be the same – that is, the avoidance of the problem food – it is important to make a clear distinction between true food allergy and the wide range of other unpleasant reactions that may be associated with food, because the severity of the symptoms and the quantity of the food needed to produce symptoms are very different. In allergy, symptoms tend to be more severe, and can be set off by minute amounts of food. People who wrongly attribute their symptoms to food allergy may be needlessly limiting their diet and their lifestyle.

This chapter explains the difference between food allergy and the other reactions to food that can occur, such as food sensitivity and food intolerance. I hope it will help you to solve the puzzle of what is causing your problems. In some cases, factors other than food may be responsible for your symptoms, and it is important to recognise and to understand this so that these other issues – which include stress and anxiety – can be addressed. Sometimes it is not easy to discover whether an unpleasant reaction to food is caused by allergy or by something else, but the effort is usually worth while.

FOOD ALLERGY EXPLAINED

What exactly is food allergy? How common is it?

An allergy to a food happens when the immune system reacts inappropriately to a substance that would normally be harmless, and causes allergic symptoms such as skin rash, itching or swelling of the tongue, mouth and throat, wheezing and even breathing difficulties and collapse. This reaction involves the production of an allergy antibody called immunoglobulin E (this is discussed in more detail in the section 'Allergy explained' in Chapter 1). If you have a food allergy, your immune system produces these antibodies each and every time you eat the food to which you are allergic, even when you eat only very small amounts of it.

Up to 20% of very young children have one or more food allergies, but most of these have disappeared by the age of 3 years. Between 1% and 2% of adults and around 4% of older children have a food allergy. However, almost 45% of the population report that at some time in their lives they have had unpleasant reactions to specific foods that they often refer to as 'food allergy'. When these people undergo allergy tests such as skin-prick testing, RAST or food challenge (see Appendix 1 for more details), most of them show negative results.

This shows up that the term 'food allergy' is frequently used incorrectly by the general public when describing food-induced reactions that are not in fact caused by allergy. Does this matter? It probably does, because if your problem is not diagnosed correctly you may not get the most appropriate and effective treatment for it. However, it might be that the only suitable treatment for your symptoms is to avoid the food that is affecting you, in which case it probably doesn't matter which term you choose to use.

If my symptoms are not due to a true food allergy, then what is causing them?

Apart from the type of food allergy that gives you the classic pattern of skin, mouth or wheezing symptoms within a minute or two of eating the food, there are a number of different ways in which foodstuffs can produce unpleasant reactions.

- **Other immunological disorders** A number of bowel diseases are caused by other disorders of the immune system, which make it produce antibodies other than immunoglobulin E (there is more information about antibodies in the section 'Allergy explained' in Chapter 1). They include coeliac disease, which is discussed later in this chapter.

- **Food intolerance** If you are intolerant to a foodstuff, you develop symptoms after eating it because your body cannot adequately handle it. This is usually because your body does not produce enough of the particular enzyme that is required for you to digest the food properly. For example, many Asian people feel ill after drinking even a small amount of alcohol because they lack the enzyme that breaks down the byproducts of alcohol. Similarly, some people cannot digest milk and milk products properly because they do not produce enough of the enzyme, lactase, that breaks down cow's milk. For them, cow's milk in any form causes crampy abdominal pain and diarrhoea. These two problems are not allergic in nature, and they do not occur if only small quantities of the substance in question are consumed.

- **Food sensitivity** Some people find that an existing medical problem can be triggered by eating certain foods: they are then said to be sensitive to those foods. For example, some migraine sufferers find that red wine or cheese will provoke their headaches. Sufferers from irritable bowel syndrome (a problem that causes abdominal discomfort, diarrhoea and constipation) find that certain foodstuffs can make their problem worse. However, these foodstuffs are not the only cause of the problem in question, and these reactions are not allergies.

- **Food poisoning** This occurs when food contaminated with germs (bacteria or viruses) is eaten. Vomiting, diarrhoea and abdominal pain result.

- **Food aversion** When someone has had a previous unpleasant reaction after eating a certain food, they may believe they will have the same reaction if they eat the food again. They may feel unwell if they even think of the food in question. Because of this, they avoid that food. This is called food aversion.

- **Other possibilities** A great many people experience a wide range of unpleasant symptoms, which they themselves attribute to certain foodstuffs. Using the tests currently available, it is possible to determine in most cases whether a true food allergy is responsible or if the symptoms are due to a particular medical disorder. However, even if the tests show that neither of these possibilities is the correct answer, it does not mean that the person is imagining their symptoms. There is a great deal that we still do not know about how the body works, and a large number of other factors – stress in particular – may be responsible.

Blaming food allergy for all unpleasant symptoms caused by foods, without proper medical advice, could be dangerous, as your symptoms might be due to another illness that should be diagnosed and treated appropriately. In addition, if you believe that a food allergy is the cause of your symptoms, you might be tempted to limit severely and unnecessarily both your diet and your lifestyle. A balanced diet is essential for good health, and no foodstuff should be excluded from your diet without good reason. Whilst it is important that you avoid any food that triggers an unpleasant reaction, it is equally important to recognise and to understand that a number of other factors might explain your symptoms. I recommend that you see your doctor, who should be able to arrange any tests you might need, and help you sort out the causes of your problem.

I am sure that I am allergic to a number of foods, including sugar, wheat and several food colourings, but my GP does not agree. He has even gone so far as to describe my symptoms as psychosomatic. I am very angry about this, as I feel he is not taking me seriously, and is saying that I am neurotic. Can I organise a referral to a specialist myself?

I can understand why you are angry, as not only have you not been offered any help for your problems, you also feel insulted by what your GP has said. I doubt that he meant to imply that you were neurotic, but perhaps he could have offered more by way of explanation. I will try to fill in the gaps.

Firstly, foods associated with food allergy are usually proteins. Wheat does contain protein, but sugar and food colourings do not and are very unlikely to be the cause of a food allergy. Sugars, which come in many different forms, are found in a huge variety of foods; the most common one in our diet is sucrose. Sugars occur naturally in all fruits (where the sugar is called fructose) and dairy products (lactose). The majority of pre-prepared and convenience foods contain sugars, including sucrose, glucose, dextrose and maltodextrin. To avoid all foodstuffs containing sugar would limit your diet enormously so it is important for your problem to be diagnosed correctly, or you could find yourself eating a very limited and probably unhealthy diet. Your symptoms could be due to a wheat allergy, but again this must be formally diagnosed, because excluding wheat from your diet can be complicated.

Secondly, although the term psychosomatic literally means 'of the mind and of the body' (it comes from two Greek words, *psyche* meaning 'mind' and *soma* meaning 'body'), it is more generally used to describe illnesses or disorders that are caused or aggravated by mental stress. It does not mean that you are neurotic, nor that you are imagining your symptoms. I do, however, feel that it is important that your general state of health and your lifestyle are taken into account when trying to diagnose what is causing your problem. Unpleasant reactions caused by food are not necessarily caused by an allergy (this was discussed in the answer to the previous question) and it is important for you to find out what is really causing your problem.

Finally, you ask if you can arrange a referral to a specialist yourself. In the UK, this is not possible, nor do you have an absolute right to a second opinion. What you can reasonably expect is to be referred to a consultant acceptable to you when your GP thinks it is necessary and to be referred for a second opinion if you and your GP agree this is desirable. In addition, you do have the right to see a different GP in your practice, or to change practice without having to give a reason. However, there is no guarantee that a different doctor will agree to make a referral.

I think that your next move should be to go back to your current GP and try talking the matter through again. If you cannot resolve it between you, see another doctor in the practice. If you are still dissatisfied after this, I suggest that you get in touch with your local Patient Advice and Liaison Service (PALS). They will be able to explain what making a formal complaint involves, but will probably start with seeing if they can sort out any concerns or issues that you have. You can find your local PALS by contacting NHS Direct or your local Primary Care Trust or looking in the phone book.

Why have I become allergic to just one or two foodstuffs and not to every food that I eat?

It is indeed amazing that food allergies are not more common, as the gastrointestinal tract is exposed to a huge number of substances that could potentially cause allergies. Although there is a great deal that we do not know about food allergy, the fact that it is so rare demonstrates just how efficient the gut is at handling these potential troublemakers and in preventing the development of allergies in most people.

There are certain factors that might have made you more likely to develop a food allergy. You may come from an atopic family (atopy is discussed in the section 'Allergy explained' in Chapter 1) – does any other member of your family have an allergic disorder, particularly eczema? In addition, the way in which you were introduced to food in infancy seems to be important. Ask your mother how and when you were weaned (if she remembers), as this may throw some light on your pattern of allergies.

Food allergy seems to be less likely in babies who are breast-fed, particularly if certain foodstuffs are introduced into their diet later rather than sooner. These foodstuffs include cow's milk, eggs, peanuts, fish, and wheat and other cereals that contain a substance called gluten. Current Department of Health guidelines suggest that all babies should be completely breast-fed or bottle-fed until they are 6 months old, and that other foods should then be introduced as follows.

- **At 6–12 months old** Vegetables, fruit, rice, meat, chicken, pulses (e.g. lentils) and cereals (oats, cornmeal, then wheat-containing foods such as bread and pasta), fish, eggs, yoghurt and cheese.

- **Over 12 months old** Ordinary cow's milk (i.e. milk straight from the bottle or carton as delivered by your milkman or bought from a supermarket).

Foods containing peanut (including peanut butter), tree nuts and honey should not be included in the diet until a baby is at least 12 months old, or until 5 years old in atopic families where other family members have allergic disorders.

I am allergic to peanuts and to shellfish. I hope to have a baby in the near future. Is this type of food allergy inherited?

The tendency to develop allergic problems is called atopy and it is inherited, at least in part. As you yourself have allergies, any child of yours is more likely to be atopic than are the children of parents who do not have allergies. This is discussed in more detail in the sections 'Allergy explained' and 'Inheritance' in Chapter 1.

However, whether or not an allergy develops is not simply a matter of inheritance. There are all sorts of other factors that come into play, some of which we know about, many of which remain to be discovered. Recent evidence suggests that an allergy is more likely to develop if certain foods such as cow's milk, eggs, wheat and peanuts are given at too early an age (current guidelines for introducing these foods into a baby's diet were given in the answer to the previous question). I would also strongly advise you to breast-feed your baby if possible, and you yourself should, of course, keep to a peanut-free and shellfish-free diet during your pregnancy.

Why is it that I have a severe seafood allergy yet my identical twin sister can eat whatever she likes?

You and your sister demonstrate beautifully the fact that, although inheritance is probably the most important factor in the development of allergy, many other factors also affect the process. You will both have inherited the same likelihood of developing allergies, but your life experiences will not have been identical. Something about the way you have come into contact with allergens (for example, how old you were, whether you were unwell at the time, and so on) has somehow led to you developing an allergy while your sister has not. This is discussed in more detail in the section 'Inheritance' in Chapter 1.

My doctor has diagnosed my 18-month-old son as being allergic to milk and eggs. Will this continue to be a problem for the rest of his life?

Allergy to milk and eggs is found most frequently in young children, and fortunately these conditions almost always improve with age. If your son avoids eating milk and eggs for the next few years, it is likely that he will become increasingly tolerant of them. By the time he is 4 or 5 years old he may be able to eat them without any problems. However, I recommend you do not include milk and eggs in your son's diet until advised to do so by your doctor, and I also suggest that he should be carefully monitored when these foodstuffs are reintroduced. In the meantime, you might find the advice of a dietitian helpful in understanding how best to plan your son's diet to avoid these foodstuffs; your GP can arrange this for you.

I am allergic to peanuts. Is it true that, each time I inadvertently eat foods containing peanuts, my allergic reaction will get worse?

No, this is not necessarily so. Although you will have a reaction each time you are exposed to peanut, this will not necessarily get worse with each exposure. The severity of the reaction can be affected by other factors, such as stress and exercise. However, it is important that you remember that you will experience an allergic reaction each time you eat peanuts, and as these reactions can be severe you should do everything you can to avoid inadvertent exposure. You will have to avoid all foods containing peanut (also called groundnut and arachis), all foods labelled as possibly containing peanut, and those containing peanut (groundnut) oil. Although distilled peanut oil does not contain peanut allergen because it has no protein in it, most cheap cold-pressed oils do and must be avoided.

Peanuts can also be found unexpectedly in foods that would not usually include them, so you must be especially careful when eating foods prepared by someone else. (For more information, look at Chapter 9, 'Allergen avoidance'.)

Is food allergy becoming more common?

All allergies seem to be on the increase. This might simply be because we are more aware and better informed about health matters these days. However, it does seem that there has been a real increase in the number of people with a food allergy and, in particular, allergy to peanuts. All food allergies are more common in people with a strong family history of the various allergic disorders (which include asthma, eczema and hay fever) and these are also becoming more common. Food allergies seem to occur more frequently in the very young, when allergies to eggs and to cow's milk are common. As these allergies have usually disappeared by the age of 5, though, food allergy is less common with increasing age.

It is not easy to calculate the actual number of people who have a food allergy, as it is often difficult to work out whether an unpleasant reaction to a food is caused by allergy or by something else (this was discussed earlier in this section). In addition, many people with food allergy never go to see their doctor about their symptoms. The true size of the problem will emerge as more accurate methods of diagnosing food allergy become available and more detailed information is collected.

Is severe food allergy more common in men or women?

This problem seems to affect young males more than any other sector of the population. Of over 8,000 people who have joined the Anaphylaxis Campaign (address in Appendix 2), 80% were under the age of 15 and 85% were allergic to peanut. Anaphylaxis is the most severe form of allergic reaction, and is discussed in more detail in Chapter 6.

I seem to read in the newspapers almost every day about
somebody dying from severe allergies such as peanut allergy.
As all of my family (I have three children) have allergies of
some sort, including food allergies, I am terrified by this.
How many people die from food allergies?

The chances of such a thing happening are extremely rare. In fact, the reason these deaths are reported in the newspapers is that, because they happen so rarely, they are considered newsworthy. Some figures may help to put it in perspective.

The most accurate information we have relates to peanut allergy. Only about four people die annually from anaphylactic shock after eating peanuts, although there may be further deaths that were incorrectly diagnosed. One in every 500 adults and one in every 1,000 children have an acute, severe reaction to nuts each year, yet fewer than one in a million of these reactions will be fatal. Around six people die each year from anaphylactic shock caused by bee and wasp stings (you will find more information about anaphylaxis in Chapter 6). Even people who have had a previous severe anaphylactic reaction have a greater chance of dying in a road traffic accident than of dying from their allergy. So, although it is essential that allergy problems are taken seriously, please try not to worry unduly.

SYMPTOMS

I am going abroad on holiday with a friend who is allergic to
shellfish. I know she usually avoids eating them, but just in case
she does so inadvertently, what should I look out for? What are
the symptoms of food allergy?

Most allergic reactions due to food cause symptoms involving the gastrointestinal tract (the gut), and these symptoms begin when the food responsible comes into contact with the mouth. Tingling and itching of the lips and tongue, swelling of the lips and the lining of the mouth, and nausea and vomiting are all common. Food allergies can also produce symptoms in the skin, causing either urticaria or angioedema (both discussed in the section 'Skin allergies explained' in Chapter 3), and chest symptoms such as wheeziness and coughing. All of these symptoms usually occur within minutes of coming into contact with the food.

The most severe problem that can result from food allergy is called anaphylaxis. This is a potentially life-threatening reaction that involves the whole body. If untreated, it can lead to dizziness, shortness of breath, wheezing, palpitations, collapse and a serious drop in blood pressure. It is discussed in more detail in Chapter 6.

In some people the symptoms of food allergy do not occur immediately after eating the food, but only after a delay of several hours. This type of reaction is much more difficult to recognise because the relationship between the food and the symptoms is much less clear. In addition, certain foods may make other allergic disorders such as asthma or eczema flare up.

You can see that the symptoms of food allergy in one person can be very different from those in another. They can also be different in the same person on different occasions. I suggest that you ask your friend for more information about her allergy: that way, you will know how best to help her.

When you arrive at your resort you should make sure you know where the telephones are, know how to ask for help in the local language, and learn the emergency service telephone numbers.

If she has an allergic reaction remember the following points:

- Don't panic.

- Help your friend to take the medication she has been given to deal with an acute attack. This will usually be an antihistamine but may also include an adrenaline injection (there is more information about this in the section 'Emergency treatment' in Chapter 6). Find out about her medication before you leave for your holiday.

- If the reaction seems to be getting worse and is causing her difficulty in breathing, with dizziness, fainting or collapse, call for urgent medical help.

- In the case of a severe reaction, your friend should see a doctor as soon as possible even if the reaction has responded well to treatment.

How can I tell if my symptoms are caused by a food allergy?

This is often quite difficult even for the most experienced doctor! The following factors would make diagnosis of an allergy to a particular foodstuff more likely.

- Your medical history, in particular whether you or other members of your family have other allergic disorders such as eczema, hay fever or asthma.

- A pattern of symptoms that occurs each time you eat a particular foodstuff.

- Symptoms that occur almost immediately after you eat that foodstuff.

- Symptoms that involve your gastrointestinal tract (your mouth, gullet, stomach, gut and bowels).

- Itching and swelling of your lips and mouth immediately after you eat that foodstuff.

- Symptoms that disappear when you eliminate the suspected foodstuff from your diet.

If you suspect that you have a food allergy, you should consult your doctor, because there are a number of ways of confirming the diagnosis. For example, you might be asked to keep a diary of your diet and your symptoms to see if there is a consistent relationship between the two, or you might have skin, blood or food-challenge tests to look for specific allergies. All these tests are discussed in Appendix 1.

If I am allergic to certain foods, how long after eating them can I expect to get symptoms of allergy?

In most cases of food allergy, the symptoms occur almost immediately after eating the foodstuff responsible. The most common symptoms are swelling of the lips, tongue or face, difficulty in swallowing, abdominal cramps, nausea and vomiting.

In some cases, however, symptoms may not appear for several hours. In these cases, the symptoms are more commonly those of diarrhoea, abdominal pain, wheeziness, inflammation of the nose, and itchiness or inflammation of the skin.

Every case of food allergy is different, and it should never be diagnosed (or indeed ruled out) on the basis of the symptoms alone. A number of tests are now available that can help enormously in the diagnosis of your symptoms, and these can be organised for you by your GP.

TRIGGERS

Is there a cure for food allergy?

No, there is no cure, so it is important for anyone with a true food allergy to avoid completely the food that is responsible. This may not be as simple as it sounds! Many of the foodstuffs responsible for allergy (particularly eggs, cow's milk and peanuts) are frequently used in the manufacture and preparation of foods, and their presence may not be at all obvious. You will therefore have to scrutinise all labels on prepared foods, and carefully question waiters and chefs when you go to restaurants to make sure that the food causing your allergy isn't in the dish you wish to eat.

This has been made easier by a recent European Union (EU) labelling rule implemented in the UK which requires the 12 foods most likely to cause a food allergy – milk, eggs, peanuts, nuts from trees (including Brazil nuts, hazelnuts, almonds and walnuts), fish, crustaceans (including crab and shrimps), soya, wheat, celery, mustard, sesame and sulphur dioxide – to always be clearly labelled. At the end of 2007, two others – lupin and molluscs – will be added to the list, making a total of 14 such foods to be labelled. If vegetable oil contains peanut (groundnut) oil, this must now be labelled. These improved labelling rules provide consumers with more comprehensive information about the ingredients in pre-packed foods and are particularly helpful for people with food allergies and intolerances who need to avoid specific food ingredients.

You do, though, need to be aware that certain allergens can crop up in the most surprising places. For example, at least one multivitamin liquid contains peanut oil, and almond oil can be found in brands of antiseptic creams and depilatory creams. If you have a severe allergy

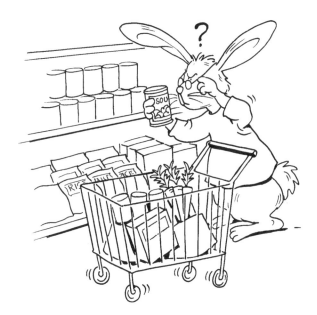

and are ever in any doubt about a product, do not use it until you have checked it with your pharmacist or directly with the manufacturer.

I think I may have developed an allergy to something I eat, but I don't know what. Which are the most common foodstuffs to trigger allergic reactions?

You are much more likely to be allergic to some foods than others, and which these are depends somewhat on your age. The commonest foods causing allergies in infancy are cow's milk and egg. Other foods, which can cause allergies at any age, include peanuts (which are actually not nuts at all – they are legumes, belonging to the same family as peas and beans), tree nuts, white fish, shellfish, soya beans, wheat, sesame, corn, kiwi fruit, bananas and citrus fruit.

Sometimes it sounds as if everything you eat can cause an allergy. Are there any foods that don't?

Foods that are less commonly responsible for allergies include the following.

- **Fruits**: apples, grapes, peaches, pears, plums
- **Meats**: lamb, turkey, chicken
- **Vegetables**: carrots, potatoes, green beans, the squash family (which includes courgettes and marrows)
- **Grains**: rice, and barley, oats and rye; however, these last three contain gluten and must be avoided if you have coeliac disease, which is discussed later in this chapter).

If I am allergic to a food, does that mean that I should never eat it?

This rather depends upon how severe your allergy is, how difficult that particular food is to avoid, and how much you like it. If your allergy is so severe that every time you eat a particular food you end up in hospital, then obviously you would be wise never to eat it. On the other hand, if your reaction is mild and perhaps limited to urticaria (nettle rash, discussed in the section 'Skin allergies explained' in Chapter 3), you will probably do yourself no serious harm if you eat the food occasionally. It's up to you to decide whether it's worth the itching! Be aware, though, that allergic reactions do not always run true to type, and a future reaction could be more severe.

The way in which a food is prepared may make a difference to your reaction, particularly in the case of protein foods such as milk and eggs. For example, some people find that if they eat raw eggs (perhaps in mayonnaise or ice cream) they develop an allergic reaction, which they do not have when they eat cooked eggs. Similarly, milk drunk in its natural form may cause an allergic reaction, whereas cooked milk (e.g. in a rice pudding) does not. This is because the process of cooking 'denatures' the protein in the food – that is to say, cooking alters it in a way that it is no longer such a potent allergen.

I am allergic to nuts – my symptoms include swelling of the lips, tingling inside my mouth and nettle rash. I have heard that if I avoid nuts for a year or so my allergy will disappear. Is this true?

No, it's not. Generally speaking, once you have developed an allergy, your immune system maintains a memory of the responsible allergen in the form of antibodies, and the allergy is therefore life-long (this is discussed in more detail in the section 'Allergy explained' in Chapter 1). The main exception to this is when an allergy develops in early childhood: the immune system is then rather immature, and its memory is not quite as good. Therefore, children who are allergic to substances such as cow's milk and eggs in the first few years of life often outgrow their allergies. However, as you grow older, you may find that your allergy becomes less active, although you would be wise to continue to avoid nuts in your diet.

I believe that the peanut is not actually a nut. Why then, now that I have been diagnosed as having peanut allergy, have I been advised to avoid all other nuts as well?

You are right: peanuts are a legume (they belong to the same family as peas and beans) and not a true nut (sometimes called tree nuts to distinguish them from the peanut or groundnut). Being allergic to peanuts does not automatically mean that you will be allergic to other nuts, although some people do have both allergies. However, peanuts are often used as a cheap substitute for other more expensive nuts, as they can be washed to remove the peanut flavour and then treated so as to taste like something else – almonds, walnuts or Brazil nuts, for example. The nut inside your hazelnut chocolate may actually be a peanut! It is for this reason that you have been advised to avoid **all** nut products, although if all your tests to true nuts were negative, it would be safe for you to eat them provided you remove them from the shells yourself and therefore know *exactly* what you are eating.

I recently had a moderately severe reaction to walnut, so my GP arranged for me to have some tests, which showed that I am also allergic to almonds. Are these nuts related?

Multiple nut allergies are relatively common, as there are chemical similarities between the different types of nut. People who are allergic to walnuts are often allergic to almonds as well. Similarly, pistachio nut and cashew nut allergies often go together. I think you should avoid all nuts, as you know for sure you are allergic to at least two specific nut types, and you could develop further nut allergies. Also, allergic reactions to nuts can be severe, and you have already had quite a bad one. Nuts can be used in the manufacture of a wide range of foods, including barbecue sauces, biscuits, breakfast cereals and ice creams, so you will need to be vigilant. Remember, too, that certain types of bean bags sometimes contain nut shells. You do not need to avoid coconut, nutmeg and water chestnuts, as these are not tree nuts and are not chemically related to them.

You should discuss with your doctor what medications you should carry in case you have another allergic reaction, as this will depend on what your symptoms were. If you had swelling of your tongue or throat, became wheezy or had difficulty breathing, he may prescribe an adrenaline auto-injector. For more information on this, see the section 'Emergency treatment' in Chapter 6.

I have had hay fever for years, but this year something new happened. I ate a fresh-fruit salad and developed itching and swelling of my mouth and lips. Since then, the same thing has happened with apples and cherries. What is the cause of this?

In certain people with hay fever, eating certain fruits can produce symptoms in the mouth and throat. This problem is called the *oral allergy syndrome*, and I think this is what is causing your problem. It is likely that your hay fever is caused by allergy to birch pollen, as people with this can also react to apples, pears, almonds, peaches, apricots, cherries, plums, nectarines, prunes, kiwi, carrots, celery, fennel, parsley, coriander, parsnips, peppers and potatoes.

The typical symptoms are itching of the lips, mouth or throat, and swelling of the lips, tongue, throat and palate. Other symptoms may include soreness of the gums, inflamed eyes (conjunctivitis) or a blocked or runny nose (rhinitis). In rare instances, asthma or anaphylaxis may be triggered. Symptoms normally appear within minutes of eating the offending food.

In most cases, oral allergy is not serious; however, it is advisable to avoid the foods that set off your symptoms. Treatment with an antihistamine will help once the symptoms have occurred.

Occasionally, people with an allergy to one food allergen may develop a reaction to foods that are closely related. This is called *cross-reactivity*. Groups of these closely related foods include the following examples:

- apple, pear, celery, kiwi fruit and peanut;

- kiwi. poppy seeds, sesame seeds, rye;

- banana, kiwi, avocado, chestnut, latex;

- barley, corn, oats, millet, rye, black-eyed peas, liquorice, lima beans, peas, pinto beans, green beans such as French beans and runner beans;

- blackberries, loganberries, raspberries, tayberries, strawberries, cashew nuts, pistachio nuts, mango;

- chocolate, cocoa, cola;

- grapefruit, lemons, limes, oranges, tangerines;

- peaches, plums, cherries, almonds, apricots;

- crabs, crayfish, lobster, langoustines, scampi, shrimp, squid.

How come I am very allergic to peanuts but not to any other members of the legume family?

Although there are chemical similarities between foods in the same food group, no two foods have exactly the same chemical structure. It is therefore possible to be allergic to one food but not to another with a similar but not identical chemical make-up. For example, by no means all people with peanut allergy react to other legumes – in fact, this is relatively unusual. There is no need to avoid the other foods in a food group if you have only ever reacted to one of them.

My child is allergic to milk. Can he eat beef?

Yes, he should have no problem eating beef. The proteins found in milk are not found in the muscle tissue of beef, which can therefore be eaten without provoking an allergy. Similarly, if you are allergic to eggs there is no need to avoid chicken.

My baby daughter is allergic to eggs. I am concerned about her having the MMR vaccine, which I believe is grown using egg. Will this be a problem?

If your child is truly allergic to hen's egg, and this has been confirmed by skin-prick testing, you are right to be cautious. Some makes of the MMR (measles, mumps, rubella) vaccine can contain a minute trace of egg protein, and this can, in very rare instances, be enough to cause an allergic reaction. It would be sensible to make sure that your doctor knows that your daughter is allergic to egg so that he can check that the vaccine used is egg-free.

If her egg allergy produces severe symptoms, she will need to be skin-prick tested to the vaccine before vaccination. If no response occurs, the vaccine can then be given safely. The skin-prick testing should be done by someone expert in the technique, and the vaccination by someone trained and equipped to deal with the very small chance that your daughter might experience a reaction. This means that both steps should be done in hospital.

Please don't be put off this vaccination, or indeed any of the other vaccinations offered to small children, as none of the other vaccines contains egg protein. In the case of the MMR vaccine, even taking into account her egg allergy, the risks to your daughter of the vaccination are very much smaller than those she would be facing if she were to catch measles, mumps or rubella.

DIAGNOSIS

I think I am allergic to preservatives and food colourings, which seem to make me moody and tired. How should I go about finding out if I'm right and which of them is the problem?

I think it is unlikely that your symptoms are due to a true food allergy, so it seems likely that you are reacting in some other way to food colourings and preservatives. It is hard to believe that all those E numbers can be good for us!

Product labelling has improved a great deal over recent years, and you will now find it far easier than it used to be to see which food-stuffs contain which E numbers. In addition, information about which additives are found in which foods is available from all the major supermarkets. You may find leaflets about them in your local branch, or you may need to write to the head office for them (your local branch will be able to give you the address).

I think your first step should be to avoid all food colourings and preservatives for a period of two weeks by eating only fresh food that you prepare yourself, and to see whether your symptoms improve. If they do, it would be worthwhile asking your doctor for a referral to a dietitian, who might be able to identify the culprits and to give you advice on avoiding them. If your symptoms are unchanged during this trial period, you should arrange to see your doctor for a thorough check-up, as other problems such as anaemia can cause the type of symptoms you are experiencing.

I think that eating milk and eggs makes my 3-year-old son's eczema worse. I don't want to change his diet unless it will be worthwhile, so how can we prove this?

You are very wise to want to find out whether or not your son is allergic to milk and eggs before you exclude them from his diet. At his age they are an important part of his diet, and it could be bad for his overall health, as well as being time-consuming for you, to exclude them unless absolutely necessary.

I suggest that you arrange to see your doctor, who will be able to advise on the best way to find out whether your son has a food allergy. The following tests are discussed in more detail in Appendix 1.

- **Skin-prick testing** This is the most commonly used allergy test. It takes only about 15 minutes and may provide very useful information.

- **RAST** This can be a more accurate test than skin-prick testing but it does involve taking a blood sample.

- **Symptom diary** Also called a food diary, this is simply a record of what your son eats and how bad his eczema is; it is used to see if there is any relationship between the two. It might be worthwhile starting this two weeks before you go to see the doctor and taking it with you.

Sometimes the only way to see whether a particular foodstuff is making a condition like eczema worse is to exclude it from the diet and see what happens. However, when children are involved, this should be done only under medical supervision, and with the help of a dietitian. If you were to exclude whole food groups from your son's diet without proper advice, he could end up eating too little of some of the foodstuffs that are essential for his good health and his proper growth.

I think I am allergic to something in my diet, as I keep on getting swollen lips and nettle rash on my body, but neither my doctor nor I can work out what food is responsible. What can I do?

Diagnosing food allergy can be extremely difficult, especially if you have no clues as to what is causing the trouble. I think your first step should be to ask your GP to refer you to an allergy specialist. While you are waiting to see the specialist, keep a food diary (also called a symptom diary). The diary should be a detailed record of everything that you eat over a period of several weeks, and you should also note down any symptoms you have during that time. Comparing your diet and your symptoms will give the specialist useful clues to the possible cause of your problems.

Your GP may already have arranged for you to have skin-prick tests or blood tests to see if these will help identify the allergen responsible, but, if not, the specialist will be able to do this. However, these tests do not always give you the answer, as a positive skin test can sometimes be produced by a food that does not cause symptoms when eaten, and blood tests are not always 100% accurate.

Your specialist may then suggest an elimination diet (sometimes called an exclusion diet). Under your doctor's supervision, you would remove from your diet those foods likely to be the culprits, to see if your symptoms disappear. If they do, you then reintroduce the foods one at a time, with an interval of at least three days between each food. If your symptoms reappear after introducing a particular food, you have found the cause of your problem.

The final stage of diagnosis is to perform a food challenge. The most accurate way to do this is so that neither you nor the person performing the tests knows which foodstuff you are being given at any particular time: this means that the results of the challenge cannot be prejudiced by the expectations of either one of you. This is done by encasing both the food in question and a harmless substance in gelatine capsules and giving them to you in random order. If no reaction occurs when you take the food capsule, that food cannot be blamed for your allergic symptoms. On the other hand, if your symptoms of nettle rash and swollen lips come on after eating a particular food (even though you didn't know you were eating it, because of its disguised form), you are sure to have found the cause. Food challenges are performed in hospital because there is a small risk that you could have a serious allergic reaction.

All the tests mentioned here are discussed in more detail in Appendix 1.

I recently experienced a severe allergic reaction to a food that we haven't, as yet, identified. My GP wants to arrange allergy testing for me but I am frightened that I might react badly to the skin-prick tests. Are they safe?

Skin-prick testing (explained in detail in Appendix 1) is part of the standard investigation of an allergic problem, and the more severe that problem, the more important it is that the cause be identified. The tests are safe and painless, although a positive reaction will produce an itchy red bump (weal) on your forearm, which can last for an hour or so.

It is extremely unlikely that you will have a dangerous reaction to skin-prick testing. If you do (this is very rare), please be reassured that the person performing the test will have available to them all the resources necessary to treat the reaction immediately, so that you will come to no harm. This is why allergy tests are performed either in hospital or in your doctor's surgery.

My daughter was recently skin-prick tested to a number of different substances when she attended the asthma clinic at our local hospital. I was surprised to see that she had a positive reaction to testing with egg, as she has never shown any signs of egg allergy. Does this mean that she now has to avoid eating eggs?

If we skin-prick tested the whole population of the UK, we would find that approximately 40% showed at least one positive reaction to an allergen, although only one-third of these people would have clear-cut symptoms of allergy. It is not surprising that your daughter had a positive skin test, as most people with asthma also have the tendency towards allergy that we call atopy (for more information about this, see the sections 'Allergy explained' in Chapter 1 and 'Asthma and allergy' in Chapter 2). Provided that she has never had symptoms suggestive of allergy after eating eggs and that her asthma is well controlled, I suggest that she should continue to eat a full, normal diet.

There is more information about skin-prick tests in Appendix 1.

When he was 9 months old, my son became very swollen around the face and had wheezy breathing after eating food containing peanut. Since then we have avoided peanut completely in his food. He is now 2 years old. My GP has suggested that we now try him with a small amount of peanut butter to see if he really is allergic to peanuts. Do you think that this is a safe thing to do?

No, it's not safe. Allergy to peanuts often appears in early life, and for most people it remains a life-long problem. In one study, for many years doctors kept track of a group of people who had peanut allergy; all of them were still allergic to peanuts 16 years after they were first diagnosed. Although young children are more likely than adults to grow out of their peanut allergy, we cannot predict who will be the lucky ones. Because of this, I suggest that you continue to exclude peanut from your son's diet. If at some time in the future you or your doctor want to find out if he is still allergic to peanut, skin-prick testing would be the first step. If this was negative, the next step would be a formal food challenge with peanut. This must be performed in hospital because of the small but real risk of a serious allergic reaction. Do not give your son any food containing peanut until these tests have been carried out and you have been given the all clear.

The tests mentioned in this answer are described in more detail in Appendix 1.

My local supermarket has started running an allergy testing service. Apparently a small sample of blood is taken by pricking your finger and the results of up to 12 allergy tests are sent to you in the post. How accurate is this type of testing, and is it worth the money?

Advances in modern technology now mean that a relatively large number of allergy tests can be performed on a small sample of blood – it is a form of multiple RAST (RAST is explained in Appendix 1). Provided that the tests are done by a reputable laboratory, there is no reason why they should not be accurate, but that is not the whole point. The results of blood tests like these will not, in themselves, give you adequate information to enable you to diagnose and manage any allergies that you may have, as all tests of this type must be interpreted in the light of your medical history and your symptoms. If you do indeed have a food allergy, you may need to be referred to a dietitian to learn how to design a diet free from the food in question. You may also need to be prescribed drugs for the emergency treatment of an allergic reaction if you inadvertently eat the food. Because all this can only be done by a doctor trained in allergy, I would advise you against using this service.

LIVING WITH FOOD ALLERGIES

My 4-year-old daughter has a severe cow's milk allergy, which not only gives her vomiting and a rash, but also makes her eczema and her asthma much worse. I am hoping to have another child. If I completely avoid cow's milk in my own diet during my pregnancy and during breast-feeding, will my next child avoid this allergy?

You are very sensible to think ahead about how you can decrease the chances of your next child developing allergies. You are right in thinking that he or she will be more at risk of developing an allergy in the light of your daughter's current problems. However, allergies do not necessarily run true within a family (see the section 'Inheritance' in Chapter 1 for the reasons why) and your next child could be completely well or could become allergic to something other than cow's milk. This partly depends on the degree of atopy your child inherits – something that is passed on from both the father and the mother.

It may be worthwhile thinking about avoiding cow's milk during your pregnancy and while you are breast-feeding. Some foodstuffs (and milk is one of them) can pass across the placenta to the unborn baby in the womb and can also appear in breast milk in sufficient amounts to cause a baby to become allergic to them. However, we currently have no proof that this would be effective, and I think that an allergy specialist would be the best person to help you decide whether avoiding milk is a good idea for you in your particular circumstances. It is not an easy undertaking, and if you go ahead you will need help from a dietitian to make sure that you eat a diet adequate in calcium and protein during your pregnancy.

There are a number of other ideas that you could discuss with your doctor. While you are pregnant, you could reduce your exposure to other common allergens such as the house dust mite, and cat and dog dander (the scales from their hair or fur, something like dandruff in humans), and also avoid all exposure to tobacco smoke. Once your baby is born, you could delay introducing those foods most likely to trigger allergies into his or her diet until as late as possible. The foods most likely to be responsible are discussed in the section 'Triggers' earlier in this chapter, and you will find information on allergen avoidance in Chapter 9.

I never let my two small children eat peanuts because of the danger of them choking. Shortly after I myself had eaten some peanuts the other day, I noticed that my son had developed swelling of the lips. I had just given him a kiss and a cuddle. Could this reaction really have been caused by the tiny amount of peanut from my lips?

Once someone has developed a severe allergy to peanuts, they can suffer an allergic reaction just from touching a peanut to their lip or, as in your son's case, being kissed by someone who has been eating peanuts. It sounds to me as though your son has been exposed to peanut before and may well have a peanut allergy, and he should be tested for this as soon as possible. This can be done either by a simple blood test or by skin-prick testing, both of which can easily be organised by your GP (you will find information about these tests in Appendix 1). I suggest you do this without delay, and that in the meantime you make sure that your son avoids all contact with peanut.

I suspected that I was suffering from a food allergy and, having
received no help from my GP, I consulted an 'alternative'
practitioner. He suggested an elimination diet, and I have been
eating only boiled chicken, rice and pears for about three weeks
now. I am getting very bored with this, and also quite hungry!
Is it safe for me to go back to a normal diet?

I personally feel that complementary practitioners and their skills have a lot to offer, and that in certain conditions they can provide some very effective therapies. I discuss this further in Chapter 10. However, this does not mean that they always offer the correct treatment!

In your case it sounds as if you have been subjected to a very strict exclusion diet, which will not be providing you with adequate nutrition. Extreme elimination diets should be introduced only under careful medical supervision, and usually require the help of a skilled dietitian. If your alternative practitioner has immediate plans for reintroducing you to a normal diet, by all means go along with this. If he does not, it is essential that you return to a more balanced diet as soon as possible, although you may wish to delay the reintroduction of a small number of foodstuffs if you are suspicious that they may be the cause of your problems. I think you need urgent help, so I suggest that your next move should be to go back to your current GP and try talking the matter through again. If you cannot agree on a way forward, perhaps you might try seeing a different doctor in the practice, or you could ask to be referred to a specialist.

My 2-year-old daughter has been diagnosed as having an allergy
to egg, and we have been advised to exclude all egg-containing
foods from her diet. I am finding this much more difficult than I
had thought, as egg seems to be everywhere! Do I have to avoid
all prepared food?

I am sorry you are finding this so difficult. Once you start looking, it is amazing just how many foods seem to contain egg. Most cakes, biscuits, chocolates, soups, sauces, custards, ice creams, pancakes, sweet breads, pastries and batters contain egg, and you will soon develop a sixth sense regarding which foods you should avoid, although you must always check the label as well.

When checking labels, be aware that egg can go by several different names, including albumen, ovalbumin, pasteurised egg and egg white. You should avoid all bird's eggs because they are similar in their chemical structure to hen's eggs.

You can buy whole-egg replacer and egg-white replacer that you can use in cooking. Egg can be used in cooking as a raising agent, for binding, for clarifying, as a glaze and for its liquid content but alternatives for all these functions can be found. Try using a vegan cookbook, as all the recipes will be egg-free. You might also find a vegan restaurant nearby where your daughter could eat safely and where you might get new ideas for recipes.

Something you might find especially helpful is a list of packaged or prepared foods that are free from egg. These lists can be obtained from all the major supermarkets – if your local branch does not have one, write to the head office (the branch will be able to give you the address). Having such a list to hand will mean that you will not be forced into cooking every meal from scratch. Be aware, however, that sometimes manufacturers change the formulations of processed foods. If one of your favourite standbys is described as 'new' or 'improved', check the label to make sure that egg has not suddenly been included. In your daughter's case, new might not necessarily mean improved.

Egg can be found in some unexpected products. Beware cake icing, clear soups, some medicines and some hair shampoos and conditioner, which can all contain egg.

You might find it helpful to speak to a dietitian about your daughter's diet – ask your GP, who will be able to arrange a referral for you.

My husband has asthma and when he takes his medication his symptoms are well controlled. I have recently been diagnosed as being allergic to sesame seeds and I am disappointed that, instead of being offered treatments similar to my husband's for this allergy, I have just been told to avoid eating sesame seeds. Why is this?

The only way you can make absolutely sure that you do not experience an allergic reaction to sesame seeds is not to eat them. In other words, there is no effective preventative treatment for food allergy, and the mainstay of management is to avoid the problem foodstuff. However, if you accidentally eat sesame seeds and your reactions are mild, you may well find that it is useful to keep a supply of antihistamine tablets to hand to treat your symptoms.

If your food allergy is severe, for example if it causes breathing difficulties or anaphylactic shock, you should be supplied with a drug called adrenaline. This can be given by injection from one of two special injection kits; you will find more information about their use in Chapter 6, which deals with anaphylaxis. Treatment with adrenaline is not necessary in mild cases of allergy.

In the very rare cases where someone has multiple severe food allergies, an anti-inflammatory drug called sodium cromoglicate (which is sometimes used as an inhaler in asthma) can be given in very large doses by mouth in an attempt to prevent or reduce the allergic reaction. This treatment is reserved for very serious allergies, and sadly it is not always effective.

I am allergic to peanuts, and just recently I have noticed that a large number of foodstuffs in my local supermarket have started carrying labels stating that they may contain traces of peanuts. I am confused – these are foods which I thought were peanut-free. Is it safe for me to eat them or not?

The large supermarket chains have become increasingly aware of the problem of peanut allergy, and are trying their best to make sure that people with this allergy can confidently identify which foods they should not eat. The foods that are labelled as possibly containing traces of peanut do not themselves have peanut as an ingredient, but may have become contaminated during the manufacturing process with sufficient peanut protein to cause an allergic reaction. This can happen, for example, when a batch of jam doughnuts is moved on a conveyor belt that has previously been used for peanut biscuits. There is concern that manufacturers are using this labelling as a blanket insurance policy, and that this has a significant impact on people with nut allergy, who find their choice of even the most basic foods severely limited. However, if your peanut allergy is severe, it would be safest for you to avoid all these foods. Although this disclaimer means that your choice is restricted, the good news is that you can be confident that the remaining foods are safe for you to eat. Allergy UK is working with a company called Safe To Eat Foods, which makes a number of products, all of which are free from additives, peanut and many other common food allergens. Contact details (including their website) can be found in Appendix 2.

I have several food allergies, but I love eating out. This obviously poses problems. How can I be certain of avoiding problem foods?

There is no way of being completely certain that the food you are eating is free of a particular ingredient unless you have made the food yourself from start to finish. Foodstuffs such as peanut are widely used in food preparation and often appear in the most unlikely dishes, such as lemon meringue pie and Chinese spring rolls.

Depending upon which foods cause your allergy, it might be possible to choose a style of restaurant that is less likely to cause you problems. For example, if you are allergic to peanuts, you should avoid Chinese, Thai and Malaysian cuisines, as they rely very heavily on this ingredient. Whichever type of restaurant you choose, and however careful you are to choose foods that do not contain your problem foodstuffs, you should remember that it is still possible for one dish to become contaminated with an ingredient from another.

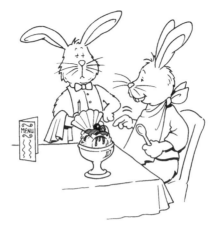

For example, meat could be cooked in a pan that previously contained fish.

Because you enjoy eating out, I advise you to become a frequent visitor to a small number of restaurants where you feel you can trust the staff to take your allergy seriously, so that you know that they will answer your questions about ingredients honestly and knowledgeably. If your allergy is to fish or shellfish, a vegetarian restaurant would be a good choice. If you are allergic to milk or egg, a vegan restaurant should be safe for you. If you have to eat out in a strange restaurant when you are away from home, choose simple dishes and, if possible, see the chef yourself to explain your allergy.

I only seem to be allergic to soya-containing foods in the summer. Why is this?

This does seem strange at first sight, but I'll try to explain it. Firstly, it might be that for some reason you eat more soya-containing foods in the summer, making what is otherwise a mild allergy flare up. Secondly, one allergy can be made worse by another: it might be that you suffer from hay fever, and so during the hay fever season you find that you become more sensitive to soya. Soya (or soy) is a member of the legume family, and can be found in many foods, including bread and biscuits, cold meats and paté, seasoned food, Chinese food (as soya, tofu or soya sauce), Japanese food (as miso and teriyaki sauce) and Indonesian food (as tempeh). It is also often found in hydrolysed or textured vegetable protein. The recent changes in the EU food-labelling laws have made it much easier to identify packaged foods containing soya, as it is one of the 12 (soon to be 14) foods most likely to be responsible for food allergy that now must always be clearly labelled.

COELIAC DISEASE

My 3-year-old daughter has been getting terrible diarrhoea, and is very thin. My GP thinks that this could be due to coeliac disease. What is coeliac disease? Is it due to an allergy?

Coeliac disease is a problem of the small intestine caused by an intolerance to a protein called gluten, which is found in wheat, rye, barley and, to a lesser degree, oats. The word 'coeliac' simply means 'relating to the abdomen' and comes originally from the Greek word *koiliakos* which means 'belly'. Coeliac disease is also known as gluten-sensitive enteropathy: 'enteropathy' means 'disease of the bowel' and again the word comes from the Greek (from *enteron* meaning 'gut' and *pathos* meaning 'suffering'). People with coeliac disease cannot eat ordinary bread, biscuits, cakes and other baked goods containing wheat flour, pasta, pizza, couscous, bran and semolina. Wheat is also present in a large number of processed foods as a thickener, and may be described as starch, wheatgerm and vegetable protein.

A wheat-free diet is not the same as a gluten-free diet, in which rye, oats and barley as well as wheat must be avoided. However, people with coeliac disease can eat these grains if the gluten has been removed, whereas someone allergic to wheat must avoid all wheat, whether it contains gluten or not.

Coeliac disease is not the same sort of allergy that you have been reading about so far in this book: the IgE antibody is not involved.

However, other aspects of the immune system are involved and anti-bodies of the IgG and IgA types are found in the blood-streams of a significant number of people who have coeliac disease. You will find more information on all these antibodies in the section 'Allergy explained' in Chapter 1.

It does sound possible that your daughter could have coeliac disease. Sufferers often lose weight and diarrhoea is common, as the immune reaction to gluten damages the lining of the bowel wall, making it less able to absorb water and nutrients from the food within it.

Although a doctor may suspect coeliac disease from your daughter's symptoms and her medical history, further tests will be required. A blood test will show if there are any anti-gluten antibodies in her blood-stream, but the only way to confirm the diagnosis is to perform a bowel biopsy (as described in Appendix 1). It is very important to make a definite diagnosis in this way because treatment involves life-long avoidance of all foodstuffs containing gluten, something that we would not ask anyone to do unless it was absolutely necessary.

I suffer from coeliac disease, and am finding it extremely difficult to buy gluten-free bread and cakes that are worth eating – most of them are disgusting! Can you help?

There are approximately 146,000 gluten- and wheat-sensitive people in the UK, and happily a wide range of gluten-free foods are now available in major supermarkets, pharmacies, health food shops and other outlets to be found on the internet. You can obtain the details of specialist suppliers from Coeliac UK (address in Appendix 2). These products are improving all the time, but whether or not you enjoy them is a matter of taste and trying out different brands.

As you obviously do not like the commercially available products, one answer might be to bake your own using gluten-free flour, although it is difficult to reproduce the texture of normal bread and cakes because gluten provides elasticity and fluffiness. As alternatives you could try using rice flour, potato flour or maize flour, all of which are available from health food shops.

If you have proven coeliac disease, many gluten-free foods (including flour) can be prescribed on the NHS. Your GP can arrange this.

I have been diagnosed as having coeliac disease, but despite eliminating all wheat-containing foods from my diet, my symptoms have not got much better. What am I doing wrong?

Firstly, you should be aware that gluten is found not only in wheat but also in rye, barley and, to some degree, oats. You should therefore exclude all four of these cereals from your diet.

Secondly, you may still be eating gluten-containing foods without realising it. Many foods list starch as an ingredient – but you have no way of knowing whether this starch is made from wheat. In theory, you should avoid all foods containing starch, unless the label says 'cornstarch' which is all right.

Avoiding all these foods can be very difficult, but help is now at hand. Coeliac UK (contact details in Appendix 2) maintains a list of gluten-free foods produced by all major manufacturers. Most of the major supermarkets can now provide information about gluten-free foods produced under their own brand names: if your local branch does not have the list, write to the head office for it (the branch will be able to give you the address).

6 | Anaphylaxis

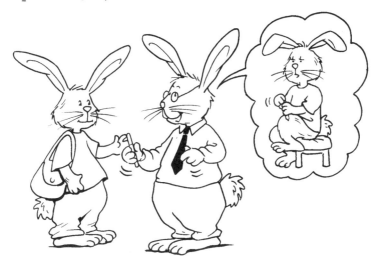

Anaphylaxis is the most severe of all the allergic reactions, but fortunately few people with allergies or allergic disorders will ever experience it. Allergy sufferers who have not suffered an anaphylactic reaction probably never will. However, this chapter should be read by everyone, as one day the information it contains may help you to save someone else's life. Each year over 3,500 people in the UK suffer an anaphylactic reaction, and approximately 30 of these die, mainly adolescents and young adults. Anaphylaxis is becoming more common, with admissions to hospital increasing eight-fold since 1995.

If you yourself have experienced an anaphylactic reaction, this chapter will give you an understanding of why it happened and what can be done to prevent it from happening again. It also gives clear instructions for the emergency treatment of an anaphylactic reaction. I hope this knowledge will help you to be less frightened by the condition and to lead as normal a life as possible. Your friends and family, colleagues at work and holiday travelling companions might also find it useful.

ANAPHYLAXIS EXPLAINED

I have recently suffered my first anaphylactic reaction. I can't remember a lot of what I was told in hospital, so please can you explain what happened to me?

An anaphylactic reaction is the most extreme form of allergic reaction. As in all allergic reactions, anaphylaxis happens because you are exposed to an allergen to which you are allergic. The body's immune system reacts to the allergen inappropriately, perceiving it as a threat. The reaction is severe, even life-threatening, and is not confined to the part of your body that the allergen touches: it affects the whole body. The most dramatic and potentially dangerous symptoms of anaphylaxis include swelling and obstruction of the upper airway, severe wheeziness, and failure of the cardiovascular (circulatory) system to work efficiently, leading to circulatory shock and collapse. If you have an anaphylactic reaction you need urgent medical attention – first aid initially, and then hospital care.

Although this type of reaction can be extremely dangerous, if it is recognised promptly and treated effectively, you should recover completely with no lasting damage.

If you have suffered one anaphylactic reaction, you are at risk of further similar reactions. It is vital that the allergen responsible is identified so that you can do your very best to avoid it in the future. Please make sure you are seen by an allergy specialist, who will be able to arrange the tests you need. I appreciate though that, however careful you are, you can never be completely sure of avoiding a particular allergen, so it is also important that you are provided by your doctor with effective emergency treatment, as described in the section on 'Emergency treatment' later in this chapter. You will have to learn how to use this treatment correctly, and so will your friends and family. You should also wear some form of medical identification to warn others that you have this problem, and this is discussed in the 'Miscellaneous' section in Chapter 8.

My friend has recently come out of hospital after an anaphylactic reaction to a bee sting. It sounds as if the whole thing was terrifying. She felt so ill that she can't remember exactly what happened, but I want to know what to look out for in case she has another reaction when I am with her. Can you tell me what the signs are?

Anaphylaxis is a sudden allergic response, which can vary in its pattern of symptoms and severity but is always serious. I am sorry that this happened to your friend, but very pleased to hear that she, like most people, responded well to treatment and has now recovered.

In your friend's case a bee sting was responsible, but anaphylactic reactions can also be triggered by other forms of insect stings, and by foodstuffs (especially peanuts and shellfish), drugs (especially penicillin and certain other antibiotics) and vaccines (particularly the tetanus and diphtheria vaccines).

After the bee stung her, your friend would probably have begun to feel unwell very quickly. The symptoms that she might have experienced include:

- generalised flushing, including a flushed face;
- a feeling of being uncomfortably hot;
- a red, raised, itchy rash like nettle rash (hives);
- sneezing, nasal congestion (a stuffy nose), itching in the mouth;
- palpitations;
- a feeling that something awful was about to happen;
- dizziness;
- nausea, vomiting, abdominal cramps;
- shortness of breath;

- tightness in the chest, wheezing;

- swelling of the lips, tongue and face;

- difficulty in swallowing and speaking;

- circulatory shock and collapse.

Your friend may not have experienced all of these, as every person's reaction is different, and the pattern of symptoms also varies from individual to individual. If the reaction was particularly severe, your friend may have lost consciousness. It is also possible that she had severe breathing problems, and even that her heart might have stopped.

All of these symptoms can be reversed by the administration of adrenaline. (This drug is also now known in the UK as epinephrine – its name in the USA.) It counters the effects of the chemicals released during anaphylaxis, and relaxes the airways, stimulates the heart and returns the small blood vessels to their normal size, effectively increasing the blood volume and increasing the blood pressure.

If your friend does have another anaphylactic reaction, the sooner she receives treatment with adrenaline, the sooner the symptoms will begin to subside. It would be very helpful if you learned to use the injector device described in the section 'Emergency treatment' later in this chapter, as your friend may not always be able to use it herself.

Which allergens most commonly trigger an anaphylactic reaction?

The commonest triggers are:

- **stings** from wasps or bees;

- **foods**, including peanuts, tree nuts, shellfish, fish and eggs;

- **drugs**, including penicillin and other antibiotics;

- **vaccines**, including tetanus anti-toxin.

Unknown factors are responsible for about 20% of all anaphylactic reactions.

Once you have suffered an anaphylactic reaction, you should assume that your allergy is life-long, and should always avoid the substance that triggers it.

I have had several bee stings in the past, but last year was stung again and suffered an anaphylactic reaction. Why did this suddenly happen?

For someone to have an anaphylactic reaction, they must have been sensitised to a particular allergen as a result of a previous exposure. In your case, you must have been sensitised to the allergen in bee venom by being stung many times in the past – but why you suddenly reacted so severely to this latest sting is impossible to explain. As yet no one knows why an allergen should trigger an anaphylactic reaction when in the past it either has caused no problems or has caused only 'ordinary' allergic reactions.

Now that you have had one anaphylactic reaction, you should assume that all further bee stings will lead to equally severe reactions. You should try to avoid being stung, and you will find some suggestions on how to do this in the section 'Living with anaphylaxis' later in this chapter. You should also ask your doctor to refer you to an allergy specialist. In the meantime, your doctor can supply you with an adrenaline self-injector and teach you how and when to use it: you will again find more about this later in this chapter, in the section 'Emergency treatment'.

My son recently had the most awful anaphylactic reaction after eating food containing peanuts. Why did the reaction affect his whole body and not just his mouth and stomach?

Your son is so allergic to peanuts that eating a food that contained them caused his immune system to react strongly, producing a huge amount of a range of different chemical substances. These substances were then rapidly spread throughout his body via his blood-stream, which is why more than just his mouth and stomach were affected. These chemicals, which include histamine, acted on the small blood vessels in his body tissues and made them leak, which in turn caused swelling. The effect of this leaking and swelling is different in different parts of the body: in the lungs it causes wheezing and breathing difficulties; in the skin it causes redness, itching and blotchy patches; in the gut it causes nausea and stomach cramps. All the organs in the body can be affected in anaphylaxis, including the heart as well as the lungs, skin and bowels.

Because an anaphylactic reaction is so widespread, enough fluid can leak out of the small blood vessels to reduce the total volume of blood circulating round the body. Once this happens, the blood pressure drops and, despite beating faster (resulting in palpitations), the heart finds it difficult to pump hard enough to maintain an adequate blood supply to the vital organs. This is why faintness, dizziness and even loss of consciousness can result. As you saw, this can happen extremely quickly, and only tiny amounts of an allergen are needed to set off this type of reaction. It is vital to recognise the seriousness of this condition and to act quickly, as you undoubtedly did in your son's case. The sooner treatment is given, the more quickly these effects can be reversed.

How do I know if I am at risk from anaphylactic shock?

You don't, until you have had your first anaphylactic reaction. We have no way of knowing which individuals will be vulnerable or when such a reaction may happen, but we do know that people who have asthma, hay fever or other allergic disorders are at greater risk of anaphylaxis than those who do not have any allergy. Bee and wasp stings are the exception – anaphylaxis to these can occur in individuals with no previous history of allergic problems.

Have you had any severe allergic reactions in the past? If you have, and in particular if they involved angioedema (discussed in the section 'Skin allergies explained' in Chapter 3), you would be wise to see your doctor. Your GP will be able to arrange for you to see an allergy specialist, who will review your medical history and advise you whether you need to carry adrenaline. The use of adrenaline is discussed in the section 'Emergency treatment' later in this chapter.

Until a year or so ago I had never heard of anaphylaxis, but now I seem to be reading about people dying from it all the time. Just how common is this?

The chances of such a thing happening are extremely rare. Severe allergic reactions are becoming more common though, and the general public are becoming more aware that they can be a serious problem. The reason you are seeing these deaths reported in the newspapers is that, because they happen so rarely, they are considered newsworthy.

Some figures may help to put it in perspective. We know that in the UK between four and eight people die each year from anaphylactic shock caused by bee and wasp stings, about the same number from food-induced anaphylaxis, and approximately ten from drug-induced reactions. In a year, only about four people die from anaphylactic shock after eating peanuts, although there may have been one or two further deaths that were incorrectly diagnosed as due to another cause. Although this is a small number, it is still too many, as every death from anaphylaxis is potentially preventable.

Greater public awareness about the causes and the treatment of this problem is essential if such deaths are to be prevented, so the media coverage is perhaps no bad thing. However, it is important to keep worries about the risks in proportion. Although each death is tragic for the family concerned (especially as young fit people are generally those affected), in reality they are still very rare. Even people who have had a previous severe anaphylactic reaction have a greater chance of dying in a road traffic accident than of dying from their allergy.

Could cot-death be due to anaphylaxis?

The cause of cot-death (the medical name is 'sudden infant death syndrome', sometimes abbreviated to SIDS) is not known. We do not believe that anaphylaxis is involved but allergy may well be a contributing factor in the sudden death of previously well infants, and is one of the many possible causes under investigation. Although we still do not know why cot-death happens, thankfully the number of cases has fallen by over one-third since 1994. This is since parents have been advised to encourage their infants to sleep on their backs, not their fronts.

EMERGENCY TREATMENT

My 12-year-old son was admitted to hospital recently with an anaphylactic reaction caused by a wasp sting. When he left hospital we were given an adrenaline emergency kit and told what to do in case it happens again. But I was so relieved that he was better that I don't think I took in all the first aid instructions properly. Please can you tell me what I'm supposed to do?

I am glad to hear that your son has recovered. You had a frightening experience, so it is not surprising that you did not take in everything you were told at the time. I hope you both never have to go through it again, but the following advice will be helpful if you do.

Firstly, ask your GP to refer your son to an allergy specialist, who will be able to confirm the diagnosis and advise about further management.

The most effective way to prevent your son having a similar reaction in the future is for him to avoid being stung again by a wasp, and there is advice on this in the section on 'Living with anaphylaxis' later in this chapter. However, it is impossible to completely eliminate the risk of wasp stings, which is why your son must carry his injectable adrenaline with him at all times. He should learn how to give himself the injection, as it is possible that he could be stung when alone. It is also important that several members of your family and some of the teachers at his school know how to give the injection, just in case he is unable to do it for himself.

If your son is stung by a wasp again and begins to develop symptoms, this is what you must do.

- Try to stay calm.

- Give your son a dose of injectable adrenaline according to the instructions. (See the next answer for more details.) I suggest that you familiarise yourself with these now by reading the instruction leaflet with the kit, and by asking your doctor or nurse about anything you do not understand. The allergy clinic will have training injector pens with no drug inside to help you learn the injection technique.

- Get immediate medical help by dialling 999 and asking for an ambulance. Give precise details of where you are, and tell the ambulance control centre that your son is known to have anaphylactic reactions and carries adrenaline, so that they understand that the problem is serious.

- While you are waiting for the ambulance to arrive, get your son to lie down and raise his legs, as this will help to maintain his blood pressure.

- If your son becomes unconscious, turn him on his side and put him in the recovery position (see Figure 11).

- Even if your son seems to recover after receiving the adrenaline injection, he must still go to hospital for further assessment and treatment. The adrenaline only buys you time by temporarily reversing some of the life-threatening effects of the severe allergic reaction – it is not a complete treatment in itself. He may need further treatment with corticosteroids, antihistamines, oxygen and intravenous fluids.

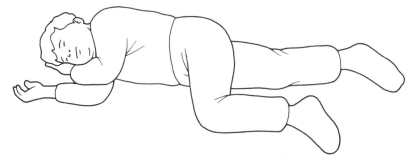

Figure 11 The recovery position

- As its effect lasts for only 10–30 minutes, your son might need a second dose of adrenaline before reaching hospital. His emergency treatment pack should contain two injector devices because they contain only one dose of adrenaline each.

- He will be observed in hospital for at least 4 hours to ensure that the reaction does not progress.

Do not delay in doing any of these things. It is far better that you give the adrenaline too early rather than too late. There will be no harmful effects if you give a dose of adrenaline when it is not strictly necessary, so administer it if you think your son is beginning to have a severe reaction. Do not wait until you are sure, as that could be too late. In most of the recent deaths from anaphylaxis in the UK, adrenaline has either not been given at all or has not been administered in time.

Make sure that you periodically check the expiry date on the adrenaline emergency kit, to make sure that it is still in date. However, in an emergency, out-of-date adrenaline won't do any harm and will be better than no adrenaline at all.

It is possible that your son was also given some tablets to take in the case of another severe reaction. These could be antihistamines or corticosteroids. Neither of these, alone or in combination, will be effective enough to treat a severe reaction and, in any case, they take too long to work: your son must get used to the fact that he will need treatment with adrenaline if ever he is stung by a wasp again, and must carry his emergency treatment pack with him at all times. It would also be a good idea to get him an item of medical identification jewellery. These are available as 'dog tags' and Velcro sports bands in camouflage colours as well as the more conventional bracelets. You can find information about this in the 'Miscellaneous' section of Chapter 8.

How should I use the EpiPen? And does adrenaline have to be injected? I hate needles.

Yes, in anaphylaxis adrenaline can only be given by injection. This is currently the only effective way of administering adrenaline for the treatment of severe allergic reactions.

Try to remember that adrenaline injections can be life-saving. The idea of giving yourself an injection is very much worse than the reality, and with a little practice most people overcome their fears.

The injection many doctors prescribe is the EpiPen. The EpiPen is available on prescription and is distributed by ALK–Abelló. A relatively new adrenaline injection kit, called the Anapen, is also available on prescription. It is manufactured and distributed by UCB Pharma Ltd. Both injectors are made in two different doses, the lower dose for children and the higher for adults. Both companies provide trainer pens for practice purposes. (Their contact details are in Appendix 2.)

The EpiPen (shown in Figure 12) is the more commonly prescribed adrenaline injection. It is very easy to use. It has a pre-filled syringe, and the needle is spring-loaded, which means that you can't see it when you look at the device. To use it you do the following:

- take the EpiPen from its carrying case;

- grasp it in your hand, forming a fist round the device, with the black tip facing down;

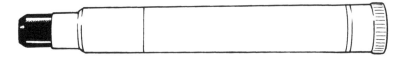

Figure 12 The EpiPen

- pull off the grey safety cap with your other hand;

- *never put your fingers, thumb or hand over the black tip*;

- let your arm hang down and position the black tip against your upper outer thigh (it is not necessary to remove your clothing unless it is very thick and bulky);

- swing the pen away from your leg, then jab the pen against your thigh firmly until you hear it click;

- hold the pen in place for 10 seconds;

- call 999 *immediately*, tell the controller that you are having an anaphylactic reaction and ask for an ambulance urgently;

- if your symptoms do not improve, or if, having improved, they start to get worse again, give yourself a second injection of adrenaline – remember to carry *two* EpiPens with you at all times.

Below are some tips for caring for your device:

- Keep the device in the plastic tube it came in. Do not put anything else (e.g. the patient information leaflet that comes with it) into the tube, because this might make it difficult to get the pen out of the tube when you need it.

- Check the expiry date regularly, and get replacements from your doctor before the pens expire. However, in an emergency, out-of-date adrenaline is very much better than none at all.

- Keep your devices at room temperature.

- Avoid extremes of heat (such as in a car in the summer) and cold. Exposure to cold may make the pen malfunction. Heat can degrade the adrenaline and turn it brown.

- If you have an EpiPen, regularly check the colour of the adrenaline in the pen via the viewing window. It should be clear and colourless. If it looks brown or a red flag is showing, it will be ineffective. Get the pen replaced straight away.

- If you use one of your devices, make sure you get a replacement straight away.

Other helpful tips:

- Ask your doctor to prepare a written emergency treatment plan for you.

- Teach your family and friends how to follow this plan.

- Make sure you have your mobile phone with you at all times.

- Practise with a dummy device until you feel confident.

- Ask the practice nurse for a refresher session if you haven't had to use your device for a while.

- Get yourself a piece of medical identification jewellery (see the 'Miscellaneous' section of Chapter 8 for details).

For more information on the EpiPen and the Anapen, visit their websites (details in Appendix 2).

Can an adrenaline injection do me any harm?

Adrenaline is a hormone (a 'chemical messenger') that we all produce in our bodies every time we exercise, are under stress or are frightened. It is responsible for the 'fight or flight' response. Adrenaline has been used as a drug for over 100 years, and it was once widely used in the treatment of asthma attacks. Because of its long history, it is a very well-understood drug and we know that it is safe and very reliable.

I don't know your personal details, but unless you are very elderly or have a heart condition, there is no need for you to be worried about the side effects of an adrenaline injection. In a fit and well person, all it will do is to push your heart rate up to the sort of level it would reach if you had just been playing sport, and may make you feel a little anxious or nervous. However, in someone having an anaphylactic reaction, a dose of adrenaline could be enough to save their life.

> *I recently had a nasty reaction to shellfish: my lips and tongue became very swollen and I felt faint and very wheezy, and I was treated in hospital with adrenaline. I've now had a letter from my GP asking me to make an appointment to be taught how to give myself adrenaline injections. I am horrified! Why can't I use the Medihaler-Epi?*

It sounds as if you had an allergic reaction that was quite severe and extremely unpleasant.

You should now avoid shellfish, but, in case you have a similar reaction in the future, your doctor has prescribed an adrenaline injection device for emergency treatment of your symptoms.

You will have to be taught how to use the adrenaline injection. I can understand if you feel frightened, but please be reassured that using an adrenaline injection kit is not the same as giving an injection with a syringe and a needle.

You should use your adrenaline injection as soon as you experience any of the symptoms that suggest you might be getting another severe allergic reaction. Your GP will probably have given you a detailed treatment plan, which may look something like this:

- Take one dose of the antihistamine as soon as you suspect you are having an allergic reaction. Chlorphenamine (Piriton) begins to work more quickly than many of the newer antihistamines.

- Use your adrenaline injector (EpiPen or Anapen) as you have been taught.

- Seek medical attention at once by calling 999 and asking for an ambulance, saying that you are having an anaphylactic reaction.

- If the reaction is severe, take one dose of your steroid tablets.

- Continue taking the antihistamine and steroid tablets for three days if your reaction was particularly severe.

I have been given an adrenaline injector to carry with me at all times, after suffering an anaphylactic reaction to peanuts. How do I know when to use it?

However hard you try to avoid eating peanuts, you may one day inadvertently eat food containing peanut and begin to develop a severe allergic reaction. You should give yourself an injection of adrenaline at the very first symptoms that suggest that you might be developing such a reaction. Do not wait until you are certain. It is far better to give adrenaline early (and perhaps unnecessarily) than to give it too late.

Give the injection as described above. It is not necessary for you to undress, as the injection can be given through your clothes, provided that they are not too bulky. Try not to be embarrassed about the idea of giving yourself an injection in public: most people these days have heard about peanut allergy, and will be extremely sympathetic. Once you have given yourself the injection of adrenaline, you should seek urgent medical attention by calling 999 and asking for an ambulance.

It is important that you become familiar with the equipment and comfortable with the idea of giving yourself an injection, so that when the time comes you do not hesitate. A trainer kit with no liquid inside is available for practice sessions, and your doctor or nurse will be able to show you exactly what to do.

I have had several anaphylactic reactions in the past, but the most recent reaction I had responded very well to the adrenaline injection. Is it really necessary for me to go to the A&E department? Last time they kept me waiting for hours and I was perfectly okay.

Severe allergic reactions are not predictable, and although your next one could be minor, it could be more severe. Adrenaline is a short-acting drug, and its effects can wear off after 10 minutes or so. It is therefore essential for you to be observed for several hours by medically trained staff who can assess your need for any further treatment. As you have suffered from anaphylaxis in the past, you should treat every allergic reaction you experience with great respect.

You should never drive yourself to the hospital, as there is the risk that the adrenaline could wear off while you were in charge of the car and that you could suffer a relapse. This would be dangerous for other road users as well as for you.

IDENTIFYING THE CAUSE

Do bee and wasp stings always cause anaphylactic reactions?

No. Only a small minority of people (fewer than 1%) will ever develop this form of severe reaction. Everyone who is stung by a wasp or a bee will experience some discomfort at the site of the sting, and this can vary from a small amount of swelling with redness and tenderness to quite extensive swelling with considerable pain. These are not symptoms of an allergy, but occur because the sting contains an irritant.

First aid is usually all that is needed – the following points are useful to remember if you are stung.

- Keep calm and, if possible, do not run as this will increase the absorption of the allergen and may make the allergic reaction more severe.

- If you were stung by a bee, the sting will usually remain embedded in your skin (wasps do not leave their stings behind). Try to remove the sting with tweezers without squeezing the poison sac (a dark pouch at the back of the sting).

- Keep the affected part cool and, if possible, apply an icepack (make sure the ice is covered by several layers of fabric such as a towel so as not to burn the skin).

- If the pain is considerable, take a mild painkiller such as aspirin, paracetamol or ibuprofen.

- If the swelling is severe, take an antihistamine (available from a pharmacist).

An anaphylactic reaction cannot occur the first time you are stung, but may occur on any subsequent sting. Once you have developed anaphylaxis, however, you will always experience a serious reaction if stung again, and so you should try, wherever possible, to reduce your risks of being stung. There are some suggestions on how you can do this in the section on 'Living with anaphylaxis' later in this chapter.

I have now had two anaphylactic reactions to peanuts. Am I likely to react in a similar way to anything else?

You would be extremely unlucky if you did. Most people who suffer anaphylactic reactions do so to only one allergen, and that allergen can usually be identified. However, if you feel yourself developing the symptoms of anaphylaxis, don't waste time thinking about what might have caused it: *start treatment immediately.*

I recently suffered my first anaphylactic reaction to peanuts contained in a dessert. Why, if my doctor knows what caused this reaction, do I now have to go through a load of tests?

It is useful to know the cause of any allergy, because this makes management of the problem so much easier. This is particularly true of anaphylaxis. You and your doctor need to be 100% confident about the cause of your reaction, so that you can do everything possible to avoid any further exposure. After all, the dessert you ate probably contained other things besides peanuts, and any one of them might have been the culprit.

The tests, described below, which your doctor will arrange are completely safe and really quite simple. You will find more information about all of them in Appendix 1.

- **Skin-prick testing** You will be tested with a range of allergens, including peanut. A positive response to the peanut allergen does not necessarily identify peanut as the culprit, but a negative test would rule it out.

- **RAST** A small sample of blood is examined for specific allergy antibodies. If peanut was the cause of your reaction, you are likely to show a positive result from this test.

- **Challenge test (oral provocation test)** Most allergy clinics no longer perform challenge tests for the diagnosis of anaphylaxis because they can be dangerous, and adequate information can usually be obtained from other forms of tests. However, if your skin-prick test and RAST both gave negative results as far as peanut was concerned, a specialist might decide on a challenge test. This would be done very cautiously, in a different way from that used for diagnosing non-anaphylactic food allergy (the double-blind food challenge test described in Appendix 1). The specialist would begin by putting a small amount of peanut on your lip, and would then wait 15 minutes to see if there was any reaction. A similarly small amount of peanut would then be placed in your mouth and your reactions observed for 15 minutes. Increasing amounts of peanut would then be put in your mouth, again with a wait of 15 minutes between each step. If this test was completely negative, you could be sure that peanut was not the cause of your reaction, and the true cause could then be tracked down.

An added advantage of skin-prick tests and RAST is that other allergies are sometimes associated with peanut allergy (such as walnut allergy), and these will also be identified.

My son recently suffered an anaphylactic reaction for the first time after eating in a Chinese restaurant. We had chosen a wide range of dishes, including a fish dish, so we have no idea what it was that caused his reaction. I am now incredibly nervous about giving him anything other than very plain and simple food to eat. How can we find out what caused his reaction?

The most likely foodstuffs to have caused his reaction are peanut (which is found frequently in Chinese and other Asian food), tree nuts, shellfish (which might have been contained in the fish dish or in fried rice) and white fish.

It is vital that your son be seen by an allergy specialist so that he can undergo a full range of tests to diagnose his allergy. He will have skin-prick tests and RAST (both of which are described in Appendix 1), and from these it should be possible to pinpoint the culprit. In the meantime it is important that he has an emergency treatment plan including the use of injectable adrenaline drawn up by his doctor, and that he keeps this treatment to hand at all times in case he has a further reaction (the use of adrenaline was described in the previous section, 'Emergency treatment').

Please ask your GP to arrange a referral to an allergy specialist as soon as possible.

I saw my doctor write 'idiopathic anaphylaxis' on my medical notes. What does this mean?

Usually the cause of anaphylaxis is obvious, as the reaction follows an insect sting, the administration of a drug to which you are allergic, or it comes on after eating a particular food. However, in your case your doctor has been unable to identify what caused your anaphylactic reaction, and the trigger remains a mystery. Hence the description 'idiopathic', which simply means 'of unknown cause' (it comes from two Greek words: *idios* meaning 'own' and *pathos* meaning 'suffering'). This puts you in a very difficult situation, as you know that you have a severe problem but do not know what causes it.

It is essential that you do two things.

Firstly, make sure that your doctor prepares an emergency treatment pack, including two adrenaline injection kits (e.g. EpiPens or Anapens), which you must carry with you at all times. You should treat any future reaction as early as possible (you will find more information about this in the previous section, 'Emergency treatment'). Once you have given yourself an injection of adrenaline, you should always seek emergency medical attention.

Secondly, you should make a very careful record of all the possible trigger factors with which you came into contact in the hours before your reaction. The interval between exposure to the trigger and the onset of the reaction is usually short but can vary between less than a minute to several hours. This information may make it possible for the trigger to be identified.

I hope that you do not suffer any more severe reactions in the future. However, if you do, their cause may become clearer and the trigger therefore easier to avoid.

I have an allergy to shellfish. In the past any reaction that I have had has been relatively mild, and confined to a little swelling of my lips and some tingling in my mouth. I have to admit that I have not been scrupulous about avoiding seafood. The other day I finished a small quantity of my flatmate's Chinese takeaway and then went out for a long run. The next thing I remember I was in hospital having had a severe anaphylactic reaction. Why did this happen, and should I expect all future reactions to be this severe?

It sounds as if you suffer from a relatively unusual problem called *food-dependent exercise-induced anaphylaxis*. Exercise can act as a co-factor (an additional trigger) in anaphylaxis: if you eat shellfish you suffer only a mild reaction, if you exercise you have no reaction at all, but if you eat shellfish and then exercise you develop an anaphylactic reaction. The exercise seems to potentiate (strengthen) the allergic reaction, although no one is exactly sure how or why this happens.

It is important that your shellfish allergy is confirmed by skin and blood tests (they are described in Appendix 1). Once you know exactly what caused this severe allergic reaction, it is vital that you avoid this foodstuff completely in the future. You will then be able to exercise without worrying that this might happen again. Although it is impossible to be sure, I think it is likely that any future reactions you have to shellfish alone (in the absence of exercise) will be of the milder kind.

LIVING WITH ANAPHYLAXIS

I am allergic to peanuts and my last reaction was severe. I ended up in hospital. How can I avoid similar reactions in the future?

As you have now had one serious anaphylactic reaction, you must assume that your problem is life-long, and do all that you can to minimise the risk of further reactions.

- **Be vigilant about all the foods you eat** Educate yourself about what you are eating and read the labels like a detective, looking for any hidden peanut. Whole peanuts are obvious, but peanut can be included in a wide range of prepared and cooked foodstuffs, and may be described on labels as 'groundnut' or by using the Latin term 'arachis'. Ask yourself what the exact source of the vegetable oil or hydrolysed vegetable protein listed on the label might be – it could be peanut.

  Restaurants can pose a particular problem, as waiters and chefs might not understand how important your questions are. You might find that fast-food chains suit you better, as they have strict quality control and list their ingredients for you to check.

- **Ask for information** Do not be embarrassed or apologetic about asking for detailed information from restaurants and food manufacturers. The more pressure we exert on them to provide accurate detailed ingredient lists the better.

- **Know about adrenaline injections** Make sure that you are completely comfortable with the administration of the adrenaline kit you have been prescribed (the section 'Emergency treatment' earlier in this chapter may help with this). Ask if you can have a dummy kit to practise with. Make sure that other people around you know how to use it. Don't be frightened of adrenaline: the dose you will give yourself has very few side effects, and is completely safe.

- **Write an action plan** Get together with your doctor and your family and write an action plan for how to handle an emergency. Sample plans are available from the Anaphylaxis Campaign (contact details in Appendix 2). Have several copies: carry one in your pocket and leave others where they can be seen; for example, in the kitchen at home and in your office at work. Check that everyone knows where your adrenaline is kept and make sure that they would be prepared to use it in an emergency.

- **Be alert to all symptoms** Give yourself adrenaline even if you have only the hint of a suspicion that you might be beginning to develop a severe reaction. Do not wait until it is too late. Get to hospital as soon as possible, making sure that someone else drives you or call for an ambulance.

- **Tell other people** Be open about your problem with your workmates, friends and family. It is not something to be ashamed or embarrassed about. The more people who know about it, the safer you will be.

- **Don't think it won't happen to you!** Despite trying their best to avoid it, approximately half of all people at risk of an anaphylactic reaction are accidentally exposed to their trigger allergen each year.

I am allergic to bee stings, and the last time I was stung I had an anaphylactic reaction. My doctor has prescribed me an EpiPen but has told me the best treatment is to avoid being stung. Does this mean that I have to lock myself indoors for the whole of the summer?

You were unlucky to have suffered anaphylactic shock from a bee sting, and I can understand that you must now be very nervous about being stung again. Try to remember that bee stings are relatively rare, and that these insects sting only when provoked. Bees are not naturally aggressive, and once they sting they die.

I would hate to think of you locking yourself away for the summer! If you heed the following pieces of commonsense advice, your chances of being stung will be small.

- Avoid wasps as well as bees, just in case you prove to be allergic to the stings of both, something that is relatively common.

- Remember that, although honey bees generally nest in commercial hives, other types of bees and wasps can build their nests anywhere.

- Never disturb stinging insects' nests or hives. If you discover a nest, call the local council or a pest control company such as Rentokil to deal with it.

- Use an effective insect repellent before spending time outdoors.

- Stay away from areas that attract insects, such as picnic grounds and the areas around dustbins and litter bins.

- Deal with any areas where pools of water collect in your garden – insects are attracted by water.

- Keep dustbin areas and patios clean.

- Get someone else to mow the lawn and trim the hedges.

- Don't walk barefoot out of doors.

- Avoid wearing perfume and any cosmetic preparations with strong fragrances, as these smells attract insects.

- Wear plain, light-coloured clothing, because bright colours and patterns attract insects.

- Avoid loose-fitting clothes, as insects could become trapped inside them.

- Keep your car windows closed if possible, and make sure that no bees or wasps are inside your car before you get in.

- Avoid drinking from an open bottle or can of drink – an insect may have flown in.

- If a bee or wasp comes near you, move calmly away.

- If a bee or wasp lands on you, don't move or try to get rid of it. Stay still until it flies away. It will not sting you unless it feels threatened.

Even with all these precautions it is impossible to eliminate completely the risk of bee stings so you should, of course, always carry your EpiPens or Anapens with you just in case. There is more information about them in the section 'Emergency treatment' earlier in this chapter. I suggest that you wear a piece of identification jewellery stating that you are allergic to bee stings; you will find details of how to obtain this in the 'Miscellaneous' section in Chapter 8.

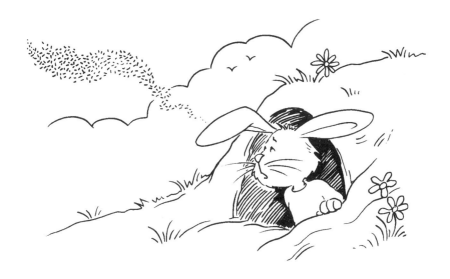

*My son has now had two very bad reactions to wasp stings, and
I am told that he almost died the last time he was stung. I am
now so terrified that I can hardly bear to let him leave the house
in summer. I have heard about desensitisation, and have asked
my doctor if he could arrange this, but he tells me that it is no
longer done. I would do anything to cure my son of his problem.
Is there anywhere that I can go to arrange desensitisation
treatment?*

Desensitisation (allergen immunotherapy) is a form of treatment
in which repeated injections of very small but increasing
amounts of allergen are given. The aim is to reduce the person's
allergic responsiveness to that particular allergen. This form of treatment was widely used in the UK in the past, but in 1986 the
government put stringent restrictions on its use because there had
been increasing numbers of severe adverse reactions, including
some deaths. It can no longer be performed by GPs, and even specialist allergy clinics can carry it out only if they follow very detailed
guidelines.

A document prepared by a working party of the British Society for
Allergy and Clinical Immunology summarised the benefits and risks
of desensitisation. It recommended that this form of treatment does
have a place but only in certain selected groups of people, including
those allergic to bee and wasp stings. So you are right in thinking
that desensitisation can be extremely useful for wasp-sting-induced
anaphylaxis. However, it is important that the potential benefits outweigh the risks of treatment; in children, these risks are greater than
in adults.

Your son has been unlucky to be stung twice, and it may be many
years before he is stung again. Even if he did undergo desensitisation
treatment, the benefits might not be long-lasting: in approximately
half of patients, the effects wear off after two to three years.

Although desensitisation is always carried out in hospital and is
always performed by doctors who are fully trained in the treatment
of any problems that might arise, there is still the risk of the treat-

ANAPHYLAXIS | 215

ment itself causing a severe reaction, which can be extremely unpleasant. This occurs in between 3% and 12% of all patients.

Each individual must be evaluated by an allergy specialist before being considered for desensitisation, but, on balance, I feel that the advice that you have received is reasonable.

Please don't despair! There are a number of commonsense precautions that you can take to reduce the chances of your son being stung again; see the answer to the previous question. In addition, he should always carry injectable adrenaline with him in case of a further sting (there is more about this in the section 'Emergency treatment' earlier in this chapter), and I think that he should also wear an identification bracelet stating that he is allergic to wasp stings (details of how to obtain these are in the 'Miscellaneous' section in Chapter 8).

The best news of all is that your son has a good chance, perhaps as high as one in two, of growing out of his allergy. I am sure that when he is older his specialist would be happy to test him using either RAST or skin-prick testing (both described in Appendix 1) to see whether his allergy has gone.

I recently suffered an anaphylactic reaction after a shot of penicillin given by my dentist for a tooth abscess. Luckily he had all the right equipment to treat my reaction, and he acted very promptly. I am now very anxious about receiving any drug treatment, especially antibiotics, and I am petrified about ever having to have another injection. What are the chances that I will have another similar reaction?

The cause of your anaphylactic reaction seems quite clear – it was the penicillin that was responsible. Further doses of penicillin could cause the same thing to happen again, so it is essential that you avoid it in all its forms for the time being. A number of different drugs belong to the penicillin family: not only penicillin itself but also flucloxacillin, ampicillin, amoxicillin and ticarcillin. They are available under a wide number of trade names, including Amoxil, Augmentin,

Crystapen, Floxapen, Magnapen, Penbritin and Timentin. You should avoid all of these, whether they are given as injections, tablets, capsules, liquids or creams.

Fortunately there are plenty of other antibiotics available that are completely different chemical compounds from the members of the penicillin family. You should not be allergic to these, so your doctor or dentist should have no problem in choosing a safe antibiotic for you when you next need treatment. There are a few illnesses that are still best treated with penicillin, but the good news is that penicillin allergy tends to wear off with time. If it was ever essential to treat you with penicillin in the future, you could be skin-prick tested to see if you were still allergic to it (this test is described in Appendix 1). However, for now you should avoid it.

You can see that it is essential for you to inform your doctor and your pharmacist (as well as your dentist) that you are allergic to all forms of penicillin. You might find it helpful to register with your pharmacy's patient database, such as Boots Medilink: your allergy will be recorded and all medications (whether on prescription or bought over the counter) will be checked to make sure they are safe for you. Your local pharmacist may offer a similar service.

7 | Allergies at work

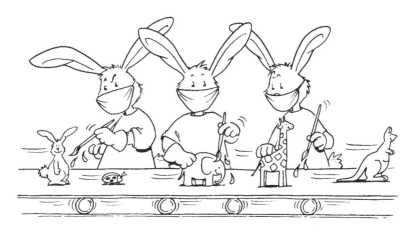

We have known for hundreds of years that certain health problems can be associated with certain jobs. For a long time, however, little attention was paid to this link, as the more onerous and dangerous jobs were done by slaves or prisoners, whose lives were felt to be expendable. The first law relating to working conditions in the UK was passed in 1802, and since then numerous Acts have followed to try to ensure that employees' working conditions are safe.

Although we have made great advances in this area, there are still a large number of health problems associated with the workplace, and some of them are allergic in origin. These are caused by contact with certain substances (called allergic sensitisers) during the working day. As you can spend about one-third of your life at work, this makes it a significant cause for concern. When investigating an allergy problem, doctors should always ask you about your occupation and your working environment.

You don't have to be atopic to develop a workplace (occupational) allergy. Although a hereditary predisposition to asthma, eczema or hay fever (this predisposition is known as atopy) makes you slightly more likely than a non-atopic individual to develop a workplace allergy, most of these problems occur in people with no previous history of allergy. It is only when working with platinum salts, enzyme detergents and animal proteins that an atopic person is at an appreciably greater risk of becoming sensitised than someone who is non-atopic.

Many of the problem substances encountered at work do not cause allergy, but act as irritants instead. This is an important distinction for two reasons. Firstly, it is relatively easy to reverse the damage and to protect workers from the irritant effects of a substance by ensuring good workplace ventilation, by wearing barrier clothing, or by replacing the irritant with non-irritant alternatives. It is much harder and often impossible to reverse the damage caused by a workplace allergy. Secondly, if you develop symptoms to a substance in the workplace, you may be eligible for financial compensation, but only if a true allergy can be demonstrated. Because of these two points, this chapter concentrates on true allergies, rather than including all the possible unpleasant reactions that may occur to substances encountered in the workplace.

Workplace allergies are becoming more common. There are over 200 known substances that can act as allergic sensitisers causing occupational asthma, and at least an equal number causing skin allergies. It is therefore impossible for me to list every single substance in this chapter, but I hope to provide you with enough general information to help you recognise whether your problem might be caused by a substance found in your workplace. The various conditions that can result from a workplace allergy are all discussed in greater detail elsewhere in this book (e.g. asthma in Chapter 2 and dermatitis and eczema in Chapter 3). Under the Control of Substances Hazardous to Health (COSHH) Regulations, employers have a legal responsibility to protect their employees from hazardous substances in the workplace, and so to prevent the development of occupational allergies. If you do develop work-related symptoms, act immediately because the sooner you avoid the allergen, the greater chance you have of being successfully treated. Workplace allergies can ruin lives. Some sufferers become so disabled that they cannot work again.

GENERAL QUESTIONS

I have heard that people can develop allergies to certain substances and chemicals found in their place of work. How commonly does this happen? Can these allergies affect all parts of the body?

In spite of extensive legislation, including the Health and Safety at Work Act of 1974 and the Management of Health and Safety at Work Regulations 1999, exposure to allergic sensitisers in the workplace is still very common. To give you some idea of the scale of the problem, approximately 900,000 working days a year are lost because of occupational dermatitis. Occupational asthma accounts for 2% of all adult asthma, with as many as 3,000 new cases occurring every year. This rises to 7,000 cases a year if you include asthma made worse by work (work-related asthma). The cost to society is estimated to be up to £10 million a year.

Occupational allergies most commonly cause allergic inflammation of the skin (dermatitis). Occupational asthma is the next most common form of workplace allergy, followed by inflammation of the nose (rhinitis), inflammation of the eye (conjunctivitis) and – rarely – allergies giving symptoms in the bowel.

What are the commonest triggers to workplace allergies?

The commonest allergens to which workers can become sensitised are:

- latex, found in protective gloves, balloons, condoms, some glues and many medical devices;

- formaldehyde, found in glues, carpeting, some fabrics, newspaper, fertilisers, furnishing foam, smoke and exhaust fumes;

- soaps and detergents, especially biological formulations;

- potassium dichromate, used in the building industry and in tanning leather;

- dyes;

- chemicals used in hairdressing;

- foodstuffs such as flour, soya, fish, shellfish and egg;

- dust from hardwoods;

- animal allergens.

Do employers have any responsibility in the prevention of workplace allergies?

Yes. Employers have a legal duty to protect their employees from hazards in the workplace, and these include the development of allergic sensitisation.

If you have developed an allergy to a substance used in your place of work, the outlook is good and there is a reasonable chance that your symptoms will disappear – provided that the allergy is diagnosed early and from that point on you avoid the problem substance. If your allergy is more long-standing, avoidance of the cause will improve your symptoms but they may not disappear completely. Because of this, all employers should aim to prevent the development of workplace allergies in the first place by identifying possible sensitisers, by assessing the level of risk to their employees from these sensitisers, and by protecting the workforce from these substances.

Employers should also provide every worker with sufficient information and training so that they can identify potential risks to health, use control measures properly and recognise even seemingly minor symptoms at an early stage. The Health and Safety Executive (address in Appendix 2) produces a large number of leaflets on these topics, which you (and your employer!) might find useful.

Who is the best person to talk to if you think you have an allergy that is caused by your work?

If you work for a large organisation with an occupational health team, you may be able to consult a nurse, company doctor or an employment medical adviser during your working hours. On the other hand, if you are one of only a handful of employees, the first person you approach will probably be your GP. Any of these people should be able to help you in deciding whether your problem is connected with work, or to refer you for further tests or specialist advice.

However, your question could be interpreted another way – you may already know that you have an allergy caused by your work and are looking for someone to help you take action to protect you from further exposure to whatever is causing the problem. In a large company with a good health and safety record, a member of the occupational health team, a safety officer, or your manager or supervisor should be able to tell you what to do next: there may well be a set procedure for dealing with work-related health matters. In a small organisation, you will almost certainly need to talk directly to your employer.

Unfortunately, there are bad employers around as well as good ones. If you are concerned that you may get a negative reaction, and you are a member of a staff association, trade union, professional organisation or similar body, you may want to approach them for advice before you do anything else. Alternatively, you could contact the Health and Safety Executive (address in Appendix 2).

FACTORY WORK

A year ago, at the age of 38, I developed asthma. This always seems to get better when I am on holiday from my job on an electrical factory production line, which I have been doing for the last 20 years. My doctor says that my asthma must be due to stress, and this is why it gets better when I am relaxing on holiday. I suspect that it might be something to do with my work, although why it should have suddenly come on after so long, I don't know. How can I sort out the cause of my asthma?

You can become sensitised to a substance with which you have worked without problems for many years. In your case it is likely that rosin (a substance used in soldering, also called colophony) is responsible for your asthma.

What makes me suspect that your asthma is due to your job is the way it gets better when you are away from work. When occupational asthma first develops, it often shows a pattern of being worse during the week and better at weekends and during holidays. As the asthma becomes more established, this pattern may continue, or the asthma may become more chronic and persist even during holidays. Occupational asthma does not tend to show the seasonal variations that are so typical of other forms of asthma. Although stress can certainly make asthma worse, the pattern you describe strongly suggests an occupational cause, which must be investigated.

Your next step should be to contact your works doctor or your employment medical adviser, who will know how to proceed. It is likely that you will be given a simple device called a peak flow meter, which measures how hard you can blow air out from your lungs (there is more information on this device and how to use it in the sections 'Diagnosis and assessment' in Chapter 2 and 'Peak expiratory flow testing' in Appendix 1). You will be asked to measure your peak flow at two-hourly intervals throughout the day, both on the days you spend at work and on your days off. These readings should continue for at least two weeks. If your asthma is due to an allergen in your workplace, your peak flow recordings will show one of two distinctive patterns. There may be a deterioration on each working day, with a rapid recovery on leaving work. Alternatively, there may be a progressive deterioration throughout the working week, with the drop in your readings being greater at the end of the week than at the beginning, and recovery taking up to three days.

If you are found to have occupational asthma, you must stop working with the substance that has caused it. You may then recover completely. If not, if you are judged to have permanently lost at least 14% of your lung function, you will be eligible for compensation.

A good start would be for you to get hold of the Department for Work and Pensions' leaflet *Industrial Injuries Disablement Benefit (Diseases)*, available from your local JobCentre Plus office, and then to arrange for your GP to refer you to your nearest allergy specialist.

I am in the process of applying for a job in a factory, and I have been asked to fill in an extensive health questionnaire. I have several minor health problems, including asthma, and I am concerned that I am going to be discriminated against on the basis of health. Is this possible, and do I have to answer the questions?

It is becoming routine these days for employers to ask prospective employees about their health, even though there are no specified medical standards for most jobs. A good employer will want to give everyone a fair chance, and will not want to lose the opportunity of taking on a good employee because of unwarranted worries about health issues. Provided that you are able to do the job properly, and that you will not be a danger to yourself or to anyone else, there is no reason why this employer should not take you on.

It sounds to me as if your asthma is irrelevant to your ability to work, assuming that your symptoms are well controlled. Even if there is a risk of becoming sensitised to certain allergens in this factory, you are not likely to be at significantly greater risk of sensitisation than anyone else, unless your work would involve platinum salts, enzyme detergents or animal proteins. It is only for these particular sensitisers that a pre-existing history of an allergic disorder such as asthma is likely to be grounds for exclusion from a particular job.

Unfortunately your worries about discrimination are not without foundation. As things stand at present, if you are asked about your health on an application form or at an interview and you do not disclose the full facts, then at any time in the future you can be dismissed for not revealing the information. At the moment there is no legal protection for applicants refused a job on account of their health (even if you could prove that that was the real reason, which is often difficult), and almost none for employees dismissed because of their health record. You might decide that you want to take the risk and keep quiet about your medical history, but a more sensible option would be to phrase your answers to the questionnaire as positively as possible and in a way that convinces your potential employer that your asthma will not affect your ability to do the job.

In the past I developed a serious dermatitis on my hands. Does this mean that I am prone to developing chemical allergies, and what can I do to avoid problems in the future?

As you have become sensitised to one chemical, it is possible that you could develop an allergy to others. There are certain things that everyone can do to reduce the chances of contact dermatitis in the future.

- Avoid materials that carry a manufacturer's skin hazard warning.
- Avoid rough or abrasive hand work.
- Avoid getting your hands excessively wet.
- Always wash your hands properly after handling any potential irritant.

- Protect your hands when working with solvents, glues, grease or oil, and corrosive chemicals.

- Avoid extremes of temperature and humidity.

- At work use any form of protection offered, including barrier creams, after-wash creams, gloves and washing facilities.

- Do not use solvents to remove substances from your hands, as the solvents themselves can cause dermatitis.

I went to my doctor recently for help and advice about some symptoms that I had put down to hay fever: I get an itchy and runny nose, red sore runny eyes, and feel a bit tight in my chest. He pointed out that hay fever doesn't very often come on at my age (I am 45), nor does it often start in the winter. He went on to ask me about my job: I work in a textiles factory using a dyeing process. Could these dyes really be causing my problems, and might I now lose my job?

It sounds as if you have an excellent doctor! He is right: although the symptoms of hay fever can start at any age and can occur at any time of year, your symptoms do sound rather unusual, and I think it is perfectly possible that they are being caused by an allergic reaction to the dyestuffs you use at work. Modern dyes (particularly a group called the reactive dyes) commonly cause allergy, which affects not only the skin and the lungs but also the nose and the eyes. Your GP should refer you to a specialist allergy clinic where you can be tested for such an allergy. Not only will they perform skin-prick testing but there is also a blood test available called RAST, which looks for specific antibodies to these dyes (these tests are described in Appendix 1).

If you turn out to be allergic to the dyes used at work, it is essential that you avoid further exposure. You should tell your charge hand, foreman, safety officer, union safety representative or works manager about your allergy as soon as possible. Your employer and the supplier of the dyes are required by law to take precautions for your health and safety. They must assess any risk to your health, prevent or control your exposure, and keep a check on any effects the dyes may have on your health. You on your part are required to make full and proper use of any equipment and facilities provided by your employer, to take reasonable care for your own health and safety, and to co-operate with your employer on matters of health and safety. You should keep all items of protective clothing and equipment separate from your outer clothing; you should wash your hands, arms and face thoroughly with soap and water (or have a shower) before going home; and you should never use organic solvents to clean dye stains from your skin. If your problems persist despite these precautions, your employer should move you to a job in which you will not be exposed to these dyes.

I am a nurse, and have been getting red, sore, itchy hands for quite a while, and the rash sometimes looks like nettle rash. I think I might have developed an allergy to the latex gloves we use at work, but haven't said anything as I don't want to lose my job. Is there anything I can take to prevent this problem?

Latex allergy is becoming much more common. Before 1979, only a handful of cases had been recognised, whereas now up to 15% of all health-care workers are thought to be affected. This may be partly due to the great increase in the use of protective gloves as part of infection precautions over the last two decades. There are other groups at risk of developing latex allergy, such as:

- Patients undergoing multiple surgical procedures (as many as 65% of children with spina bifida are allergic to latex).

- Individuals with a history of certain food allergies, such as banana, avocado, kiwi and chestnut, because of cross-reactivity between these allergens (for more information on this, see Chapter 5).

- Individuals with existing atopic disease (estimated as some 30–40% of the UK population).

- Other individuals exposed to latex on a regular basis, e.g. car mechanics and workers in the catering and electronics trades.

In the hospital environment, latex is found in protective gloves, stethoscopes, elastic bandages and support dressings, tubing used for intravenous drips and catheters, mattress protectors, rubber bungs on medication vials, blood pressure cuffs and in many other medical products. Household items commonly containing latex include rubber bands, erasers, balloons, condoms, swimming goggles and caps, underwear elastic, the buttons on TV remote controls, baby bottle teats and hot water bottles.

There are three ways in which latex can cause symptoms, not all of which are due to allergy:

- It can act as an irritant causing red, sore or cracked skin, which is confined to the area of contact and recovers as soon as exposure stops. This is not caused by allergy.

- It can cause allergic sensitisation, so that any later contact with latex causes an immediate allergic reaction, which comes on within minutes. This can cause a localised or generalised skin rash with hives (urticaria), as well as having effects on the lungs, nose and eyes, including wheezing, and redness, itching and increased secretions of the nose and eyes, rather like in hay fever.

- It can cause a delayed type of allergic reaction, which can take as long as 24 hours to develop. This is due to the chemicals (mercaptobenzothiazole and thiurams) used in the manufacturing process of latex rubber and not the latex itself, and can occur to other, non-latex rubbers made using the same chemicals. The typical skin rash is red and scaly, and occurs on areas exposed to latex. (For more information, see Chapter 3.)

It is vital that you tell your employer that you think you have developed an allergy to latex. Your symptoms are relatively mild at present, but they could become worse and there is a small risk that you could develop severe allergic reactions, including anaphylaxis, with continued exposure. If you get help when your symptoms are mild, you might prevent more serious reactions from occurring.

You should be referred to your occupational health department, where you can be tested using skin-prick testing and a blood test called RAST (for more information, look at Appendix 1). If you prove to be allergic, your employer has a duty to protect you from further exposure to latex and to regularly assess your health.

WORKING OUTDOORS

My 18-year-old son has just taken up a job as a trainee gardener. Since starting work he has developed very sore and itchy hands, with blistering at times. He is very reluctant to tell his employer or to go to our doctor as he loves the job and would hate to lose it. Is this likely to be an allergy, and what is likely to be causing it?

It does sound as if his problem is allergic in nature. A wide range of plants can start off an allergic process and cause contact dermatitis (the medical name for your son's skin problems). Among those commonly encountered in the UK and well known to cause skin problems are:

- Alstroemeria;

- chrysanthemums and various other members of the daisy family;

- Daphne (some species only);

- euphorbia;

- ivies;

- Leyland cypress;

- *Primula obconica*;

- Schefflera;

- bulbs such as tulips, lilies, hyacinths and narcissus.

A form of skin testing called patch testing (described in Appendix 1) may well be able to identify the culprit. If he is allergic to only one or two plants, it might be possible for him to avoid these completely. If not, he could make sure he always wears gloves whenever he has to handle them. Only if his symptoms persist despite these measures will he have to reassess whether this is the right job for him.

My husband is a forestry worker and, although he won't admit it, his asthma was very much worse in the autumn and early winter last year. He had some really bad attacks, and slept extremely badly. He was very much better during the Christmas holiday, when we mostly stayed at home. Was this coincidence, or could there be something about his job that makes his asthma worse?

Almost certainly the triggers for your husband's asthma last autumn were the spores produced by moulds and fungi, which grow particularly well in the dark damp conditions of a forest. I would advise him to go to see his doctor, who will prescribe treatment with adequate levels of preventative (anti-inflammatory) medications to keep his asthma under control. Your GP may also give your husband a peak flow meter so that he can keep a record of his lung function on a day-to-day basis. Your husband may require extra medication during the mould spore season, which starts in September. His peak flow recordings will be useful in showing what level of treatment he requires.

There is more information on peak flow recordings in the sections 'Diagnosis and assessment' in Chapter 2 and 'Peak expiratory flow testing' in Appendix 1, and on preventative treatment for asthma in the section 'Treatment' in Chapter 2.

OFFICE WORK

I am a secretary, and work on a computer with a VDU screen for up to eight hours a day. I have terrible problems with my eyes: they always feel tired and dry and itchy, and now my face is also red and itchy. I am sure the VDU is the cause, but my boss disagrees. Who is right?

Visual display units (VDUs) have been in use for a long time, and are now virtually everywhere. Like you, some people find that they develop sore eyes when working long hours with these screens. This is because people blink less when staring at a VDU screen than they normally do. Because of this, tears (the eyes' natural lubricant) are less well distributed over the eyes, which therefore become slightly dry and irritated. You can reduce the problem by making sure that you have frequent breaks from looking at your screen. The VDU should be positioned carefully so as not to be against a bright light or window, and so as not to reflect bright lights in the screen. A filter fitted over your VDU screen will also help to reduce glare.

There have been a number of reports of redness and itching of the face in VDU workers. This might be caused by the combination of a dry atmosphere in the workplace and increased static electricity near the VDU. Try using a simple emollient cream such as E45 (available from most chemist's) and, if the condition does not improve, arrange to see your doctor.

Finally, some people worry that they are being affected by radiation from VDUs, but this is very unlikely to be the cause of any problems. VDUs do give off a small amount of radiation but this is less than the amount given off by the average human body, which is itself slightly radioactive.

I always feel unwell at work but feel much better at weekends. Several of my colleagues in the office find the same. We think that our building has sick building syndrome. What causes this?

A few years ago there were many reports of supposed sick building syndrome, and a number of studies have been carried out to investigate this phenomenon. It does seem that certain buildings can make the people working in them feel unwell, but no one is sure why this happens. One of the suggested causes was a high concentration of the house dust mite. However, allergy to the house dust mite generally causes clear-cut allergy symptoms such as asthma, rhinitis or eczema, whereas your symptoms sound rather more generalised.

Air-conditioning (which makes the air very dry) or overheating (due to lack of natural ventilation) could both be responsible for making you feel generally off-colour. You could try getting outside for a walk and some fresh air as often as you reasonably can during the day, and see if this helps solve your problem. And have you considered whether you are happy at work, or if you dislike your job for some reason? Feeling negative about your work, which fills a considerable proportion of your waking hours, could add to your feeling unwell during the week.

I would advise you to see your doctor, who will give you a general check-up and who could also arrange for allergy testing if this seems to be appropriate.

OTHER OCCUPATIONS

I have developed bad eczema on my hands since becoming an assistant chef. This seems to be because of an allergy to the foodstuffs that I handle. Is this possible? I have also been told that I must stay off work until my hands recover, because I am putting customers at risk of food poisoning. How can this be?

It is most likely that your problem is not in fact eczema but a form of contact dermatitis, which can be caused by a wide range of foodstuffs.

People working in catering are particularly at risk because their hands are often wet and they frequently suffer small cuts: both these factors allow allergens to penetrate the skin.

I recommend that you see your doctor urgently and ask for a referral to a dermatologist (a doctor who specialises in treatment of the skin and its problems), as you cannot return to work until the problem is cleared up. The specialist should be able to identify which foodstuffs are causing the problem, either by patch testing or by using RAST (both these tests are described in Appendix 1). Once the cause of your dermatitis has been identified, you might be able to avoid contact with it – wearing plastic gloves may help. However, if the problem continues, you might unfortunately have to consider changing your career, as your employer is perfectly correct: severe contact dermatitis on the hands can become infected with organisms which, if passed on to the food, can cause food poisoning.

I am a hairdressing trainee, and recently I developed a nasty inflammation on my hands. My boss suggested I started wearing gloves, but since then my hands have got very much worse and I now can't work. What is causing this awful irritation, and what can I do?

I suspect that the initial soreness and inflammation of your hands was due to irritation from the chemicals used in hairdressing. To combat this you started wearing gloves, which probably contained latex. I think you may now have developed a latex allergy, and the more severe dermatitis you have experienced recently is from the gloves, rather than from the hairdressing chemicals.

There are a number of things you can try that might improve the condition of your hands.

- Keep your hands clean and dry whenever possible.

- Ask your employer for plastic (latex-free) gloves, which you should wear only when absolutely necessary, in order to avoid getting chemicals onto your skin.

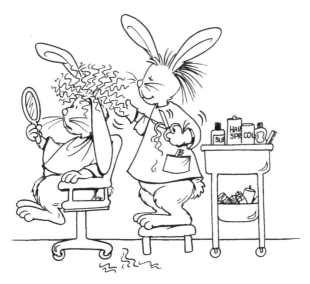

- Be very careful with anything that might scratch or cut your hands.

- Ask your doctor to arrange for you to be tested for allergy to latex as well as to the common hairdressing chemicals.

If you prove to be allergic to latex but not to any of the hairdressing chemicals, I can see no reason why you can't continue in your present job (making sure that you always use latex-free plastic gloves when you need to protect your hands). If, however, you prove to be allergic to any of the dyeing or perming solutions, you might have to rethink your choice of career.

I work in a garage. A month or two ago I developed really sore hands, and since then have been making sure that I remove as much of the oil and grease from my hands at the end of the day as possible by using a solvent. Despite that, my hands seem to be getting worse and worse. What can I do?

The first thing you should do is to stop using the solvent. Although this may seem to remove the oil and grease from your hands, using it actually allows a greater amount of these substances to penetrate your skin, and can itself cause allergies.

Your problem sounds like a form of contact dermatitis caused by one of the chemicals you use during your working day. From now on, you should try to protect your hands from all oil, grease, lubricants and fuel oils, either by wearing gloves or by using a suitable barrier cream (your employer should be able to provide this for you), which should be put on at the beginning of the day when your skin is completely clean. Try to keep your hands dry as much as possible, and try to avoid minor skin trauma such as cuts and scrapes. At the end of the day, clean your hands with a detergent-based rather than a solvent-based preparation. If your problem persists despite these efforts, I suggest that you ask your doctor to refer you to a dermatologist for allergy testing.

My 16-year-old daughter has started a Saturday job in a pet shop. She loves animals and hopes to pursue a career as a veterinary nurse. The problem is that her eczema, which she has had off and on since infancy, has got dramatically worse, and I think sometimes I can hear her wheezing. She says everything is fine and refuses to go to the doctor but I am very worried about her. Could her Saturday job be responsible? By the way, we don't have any pets at home because my husband is allergic to both cats and dogs.

I think your daughter is almost certainly allergic to one or more of the animals that she cares for at work. As she loves animals, she probably spends as much time with them as possible, stroking and petting them and so getting large doses of allergen onto her skin and into her lungs in the process.

The first thing to do is to advise your daughter not to pick up or pet any of the animals at work. I would recommend that she sees your doctor as soon as possible to ask if she can be referred for skin testing to common animal allergens such as cat, dog, guinea-pig and horse. Your GP will also prescribe appropriate treatment for her eczema, and should ask her to keep regular recordings of her lung function to see whether she is developing asthma (if so, she may require treatment for this as well). This is a simple test, which is done at home using a portable peak flow meter; it is explained further in the sections 'Diagnosis and assessment' in Chapter 2 and 'Peak expiratory flow testing' in Appendix 1.

Once her symptoms are under control and you have the results of the allergy tests, then you, your doctor and your daughter can discuss together what she should do about her Saturday job, and whether she would be wise to rethink her future career.

I was made redundant last year, and have recently set myself up as a self-employed painter and decorator. I have always been in good health until now, but over the past few months I have noticed that my chest often feels very tight and I have difficulty breathing when I am at work. Could I be reacting to one of the paints I use, and, if so, how do I find out which one?

Paints are made from a wide range of chemical substances including pigments, solvents, dryers and extenders. Some of these can act as irritants, and some of them can also be responsible for causing an allergy – as sounds likely in your case.

It may prove very difficult to find out which paint is causing your allergy, but you may find the following pieces of advice helpful.

- Use water-based paints wherever possible.

- Make sure the room in which you are working is as well ventilated as possible.

- Always replace the lids on containers to reduce the release of fumes and vapours into the atmosphere.

- Keep your work area as dust-free as possible.

- Never eat, drink or smoke while painting.

- Take care when cleaning your brushes and other equipment so as not to spray fine particles into the air.

- Wash your hands and take off your protective clothing before going home.

- Consider using a respirator fitted with an appropriate filter.

If your symptoms persist, ask your GP to refer you to a specialist allergy clinic where they might be able to identify the substance causing your allergy. You might then be able to avoid using paints or solvents containing this particular chemical.

8 | Living with allergies

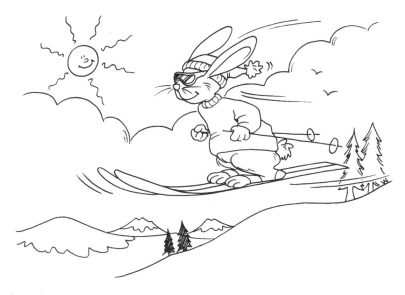

This chapter deals with some of the very practical questions about everyday matters that are frequently asked by people with allergies of all types. It covers a broad sweep of topics but concentrates on situations when having an allergy can pose particular problems. Going on holiday, going to school and being admitted to hospital (perhaps for an operation totally unconnected with your allergy, perhaps because you are having a baby) will all involve you in new experiences.

Remember that it is possible to avoid many potential hazards by maintaining control over certain aspects of your life while away from home. For example, if your child has a severe food allergy, you can send packed lunches with him or her to school, and stay in self-catering accommodation when on holiday. These strategies can reduce anxiety, which, as we know, in itself can make allergies worse. I hope that the information given here – combined with a bit of forward planning – will help you to cope better with these situations. And, in the case of holidays, to enjoy them!

HOLIDAYS AND TRAVEL

I have never had a holiday abroad because I am too frightened
that my asthma will get worse and that something awful will
happen. Am I being unnecessarily cautious?

Obviously you shouldn't go abroad on holiday unless you think
you would enjoy it, but I do think you are probably being a little
over-cautious in not allowing yourself to try a foreign holiday at all.
You are particularly concerned about your asthma, but people with
other allergies (or other medical conditions entirely) have worries
about foreign travel that are very similar to yours. If you can work
out exactly what it is about going abroad that troubles you, you can
plan how to address that problem or what to do if it occurs.

- If it is the thought of language problems that worries you –
  that you might not be able to make yourself understood to
  people in your holiday resort or to health-care professionals –
  why not consider a holiday in an English-speaking country?

- If it is the thought of flying that worries you, why not travel to
  continental Europe by sea or via the Channel Tunnel?

- If you are concerned about the standard of medical care
  abroad, why not choose a country with a modern and efficient
  health service? You may feel better when you remember that
  asthma and other allergies are common in many countries, so
  that wherever you are (provided that you are not too far off the
  beaten track), it is likely that the doctors will be highly
  experienced in dealing with these conditions.

There are sensible precautions you can take to try to ensure that
your holiday is as trouble-free as possible as far as your health and its
care is concerned, and these are discussed in the following answers
in this section. I hope I can reassure you that, with sufficient forward
planning, it is possible for people with atopic conditions and allergies

to travel safely and enjoyably anywhere they wish to go, and that you now have the confidence to try a holiday abroad. Perhaps a good way to start would be with a short holiday somewhere not too far afield, with a tour operator who will provide you with the services of an English-speaking representative.

Can I get supplies of my usual medication in other countries if I need to for any reason, say if all my luggage is stolen?

As you do not say what treatment you are taking or for which allergy, I can only answer your question in general terms.

- Most of the commonly prescribed allergy treatments are available in other economically developed countries, but may be more difficult to obtain in more exotic or remote holiday destinations.

- Recently developed drugs may only be available in a limited number of countries.

- The formulation, strength and brand name of your usual treatment may be different in another country. All drugs have two names: a generic name and a brand (or trade) name. The generic name is the true or scientific name of the drug, given to it when it is first developed, and that name normally remains the same wherever you are in the world. The brand name is the name given to the drug by the manufacturer, and that name can vary from country to country, or from manufacturer to manufacturer if it is made by more than one pharmaceutical company.

The medical information departments of the major pharmaceutical companies will be able to tell you which of their products are available in which countries and under what names. I suggest that you check with the company making your particular treatment before you travel, and take a note of the details with you, including the generic name of your medication. In addition, take the precautions detailed in the next answer.

Before I leave to go on holiday I try to make sure I have enough medication to last while I'm away, but are there any other precautions I should take?

There are, and forward planning is well worth the effort as it will help to make sure that your holiday is a success. You may find some or all of the following points helpful.

- Choose a holiday destination that is the least likely to trigger your particular allergy. There is no best place to go, but from your past experience you may know of places to avoid.

- Contact your holiday company well in advance to ask for any specific requirements, such as feather-free bedding or a special diet. Ask them to confirm in writing that they will be able to meet your special needs, and take their letter with you when you go in case of any administrative slip-ups.

- Make sure that your symptoms are as well controlled as possible before you go on holiday. If you are at all concerned, visit your GP or practice nurse in plenty of time so that any necessary adjustments can be made to your treatment.

- Ask your GP to provide you with a written plan explaining what you should do if your allergy gets worse while you are away. For example, if you have asthma, your doctor may prescribe a course of oral steroid tablets for you to take should you need them.

- If you are travelling to a European Union country or Switzerland, take your European Health Insurance Card (EHIC) with you, as this entitles you to free or reduced-cost medical care. The EHIC, which superseded the E111 on 1 January 2006, is available free of charge from any Post Office or online via the Department of Health website (see Appendix 2 for contact details). You should remember to do this even if you are only going across the Channel for a day's shopping or a short break.

- Obtain travel insurance even if you have an EHIC, because this may not cover everything you might expect to receive on our National Health Service, and will not cover the costs of bringing you back to the UK.

- When arranging medical insurance to cover you while you are away, get good advice on how much cover you may need (health-care costs vary considerably in different parts of the world). Remember to give details of your allergy on the insurance application form – if you do not mention it, it will not be covered. (Asthma UK can help you find an insurer who is asthma-friendly; their contact details are in Appendix 2.)

- Make sure that you carry supplies of all your medications in your hand luggage so that they are readily accessible, and carry a back-up supply in a separate bag, in case one bag is lost or stolen.

- Know the generic (scientific) name for your medications because trade (brand) names often vary between countries. Because of this, it is best to keep your medications in their full packaging rather than decanting them into other containers.

- When you arrive at your destination, find out where the nearest telephone is, how to call for a doctor and an ambulance, and the whereabouts of the nearest hospital accident & emergency (A&E) department.

- Make sure your travelling companions know about your allergy and how to help you if you have an acute problem.

- Take this book with you if you have space in your luggage! It will be a source of information for both you and your companions. Another publication you may find useful is the *Traveller's Guide to Health* which is produced by the Department of Health (details of how to obtain a copy are in Appendix 3).

I worry that my medication might be confiscated when I go through customs. Could this happen, and, if so, what should I do?

If you are travelling to Western Europe, North America, Australia or New Zealand, there should be no problems about your medication, as it is unlikely to be confiscated. Allergies are common and well recognised in these parts of the world – for example, as many as 10% of travellers might be carrying asthma inhalers – so customs officers are used to seeing people who need to keep their routine medication with them.

If you are travelling further afield, it might be wise to carry a letter from your doctor explaining what your medication is for, why you must carry it, and confirming that it has been prescribed for your personal use. This might prove useful if you have any difficulties. You might also find it worthwhile to contact the embassies of the countries you are visiting to ask for their advice before you leave.

I am only going away for a short time. Would it be all right to stop my asthma treatment while I am away?

No it would not be all right! Even if you are only away for a short period of time, you should continue to take your prescribed treatment or your allergy could get worse and spoil your holiday. For example, if you have asthma and you stop taking your preventer inhaler regularly, you run the risk of precipitating a general worsening of your asthma and even provoking a severe asthma attack. As well as using your preventer inhaler regularly, you should always carry your reliever inhaler with you. It could be very dangerous for you not to have the means of treating your asthma symptoms if they occur while you are on holiday.

I have asthma. Is it safe for me to fly?

Yes. Modern aeroplanes are pressurised so that conditions inside them are almost the same as on the ground. Make sure when you book your seat that you are flying with a non-smoking airline or, failing that, that you are as far away as possible from the smoking section. If you might need to use a nebuliser on board, warn the airline when you book your seat. They may be able to provide you with a nebuliser, or will be able to arrange for you to use your own. Make sure that you take all your medications on board with you, as most airlines carry only a small supply of medications. Try to plan your journey carefully so that you avoid situations that might make you anxious or upset, as these emotions might bring on an attack. Make sure that your symptoms are as well controlled as possible in the weeks leading up to your trip, and that you get your doctor to write an emergency treatment plan in case you experience a worsening of your asthma while away.

I have been offered a promotion at work, and my new job would involve a lot of travelling, particularly to North America. I have both asthma and hay fever, so this a good idea?

Provided that you are conscientious about taking your preventer treatments for your asthma (remembering to allow for the differences in time zones), and follow the other advice for trouble-free travelling given in this section, there is no reason why you should not be able to travel frequently without too many problems.

Are there any holiday activities that I should avoid because of my asthma?

Most doctors would advise that people with current asthma should not scuba dive. This can be dangerous because:

- There is an increased risk of an acute asthma attack during a dive, owing to the increased physical exertion and the dryness of the compressed air.

- Most regulators (the valve through which a diver breathes) leak small amounts of sea water, which is then nebulised and inhaled. Salt water is a potent trigger for spasm of the small airways and can cause an asthma attack.

- There is an increased risk of heart rhythm disturbance in people using a bronchodilator.

If you have not had asthma symptoms since childhood, or have been symptom-free for two years and are not on current medication, scuba diving may well be safe. See your doctor, who knows your personal circumstances, and ask his opinion.

Other activities that are particularly exhilarating (such as parachuting) or that involve moving in restricted spaces (such as potholing) should probably also be regarded with caution. Otherwise, provided that your asthma is well controlled, and you have your reliever inhaler with you, you should be able to participate in almost all holiday activities.

Is skiing safe for an asthmatic?

The main triggers for asthma that skiing can present are:

- the air at altitude is cold and dry;
- in misty or white-out conditions, the air is loaded with water vapour;
- it involves periods of physical exertion.

All of these can provoke acute asthma symptoms. However, as long as you ensure that you always have access to your reliever medication and your asthma is well controlled, it should not prevent you from skiing.

Can I take my nebuliser abroad?

Assuming that the voltage of the power supply in the country you are visiting is similar to that in the UK (240 volts), all you will need to be able to use your nebuliser is an adapter for the plug. The compressors of some modern nebulisers have an integral battery so that they can be used independently of the mains for a while, but because these batteries have only a limited life, even these will need a power supply at some stage for recharging them.

If the voltage is different (as in the USA), you will not be able to use your nebuliser unless it has a dual voltage facility.

For more information about nebulisers, see the section 'Treatment' in Chapter 2.

I am severely allergic to peanuts. How can I be sure that I'm not given food with peanuts in while I'm on holiday?

One of the safest ways to ensure that you do not accidentally eat food containing peanuts is to prepare all of your food yourself. However, a self-catering holiday is not everybody's idea of a perfect break!

If you want to eat in a restaurant, it is vital that you are able to explain to the people cooking and serving your food that you must not eat peanuts. Use simple and direct language; for example, 'If I eat even the smallest amount of peanut, I will suffer a serious allergic reaction that could make me very unwell or even kill me.' It is important that they are left in no doubt about the seriousness of your allergy. If you are not fluent in the language of the country you are visiting, it might help to take a pre-prepared card with you, giving the necessary details in the appropriate language, which you can then show whenever you need to. You may need help in preparing the card (it is obviously important that it is correct). Allergy UK (formerly the British Allergy Foundation) and the Anaphylaxis Campaign (the addresses are in Appendix 2) produce a series of pre-prepared cards in various languages, and one of these might be exactly what you need. If not, perhaps a local language teacher could help, or you could contact the Institute of Translation and Interpreting (again, the address is in Appendix 2).

Accidents can still happen, so you must carry your treatment with you at all times, in the form of either an EpiPen or an Anapen. Make sure that your adrenaline preparation has not reached its expiry date, and that both you and your travelling companions know how to administer it. You will find more information about adrenaline in the section 'Emergency treatment' in Chapter 6.

I am very allergic to insect bites, and I'm dreading my holiday because I always seem to get badly bitten. Is there anything I can do to put the insects off me? They never seem to bite my husband!

Yes, there are all sorts of things that you can try.

- Use an effective insect repellent on all exposed skin surfaces, avoiding your lips and eyes. You may find that an insect repellent bought locally is more effective against that country's insect population.

- Cover as much of your body as possible when spending time out of doors, especially in the evening.

- If possible, avoid being out of doors in the evening, when insects are much more active.

- Wear light-coloured clothing. Bright colours and dark clothing attract insects.

- Avoid perfume and scented skin creams, deodorants, cosmetics, hair spray, etc. The smell attracts insects.

- Stay away from areas such as rubbish bins and picnic grounds, where insects are likely to be found.

- Mosquitoes breed in wet, swampy areas, so avoid areas of still water.

- If you are on a self-catering holiday, keep kitchen areas and rubbish bins clean and free from food scraps.

- There is some evidence that certain insects (particularly

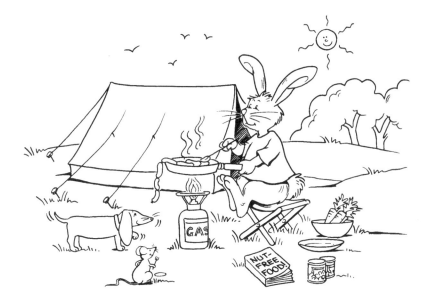

mosquitoes) dislike the taste and smell of vitamin B_1 (thiamine). Try taking 100 mg of vitamin B_1 once a day, starting two weeks before you go away and continuing throughout your holiday.

- Use a 'knock-down' insect spray in your bedroom before you go to bed at night.

- Consider using a mosquito net over the bed at night.

SCHOOL

My 4-year-old daughter, who has asthma, is about to start school. What information should I give her teachers?

The school will probably already be familiar with the problems that asthma can cause because as many as one in eight children of this age have asthma. However, it would still be sensible to provide your daughter's teachers with some written details, which should include the following information.

- The medications your daughter routinely needs to take at school.

- Details of any medications she needs before exercise.

- A treatment plan of exactly what to do if her asthma suddenly gets worse.

- Telephone numbers on which you, your partner or another responsible relative can be contacted at all times.

- The telephone number of your daughter's doctor.

- Information about things known to trigger your daughter's asthma; e.g. pets, exercise and excitement.

You may find it useful to give the school some more general information about asthma. Asthma UK produces excellent information packs for schools.

Every school should now have its own asthma policy, which will probably be based on the one suggested by Asthma UK. The Department for Education and Skills also produces guidelines for the management of asthma in schools. Contact details for these organisations can be found in Appendix 2. With the help of this information, your daughter's teachers should feel well equipped to cope with her asthma.

I have three children and they all have allergies, although only one of them has asthma. I assume the sort of information I give their teachers will be much the same for all of them, but do schools know as much about other allergies as they do about asthma?

You are right; the information that teachers need is much the same, whatever a child's allergy. You could use the list in the previous answer as a starting point, simply adapting it where necessary to cover each child's particular needs. However, although all schools should now have an asthma policy, the same is not true of other allergy problems, so they will probably appreciate extra information about your children's particular allergies. As well as specific instructions about each of your children, why not offer the school some of the leaflets produced by Allergy UK (formerly the British Allergy Foundation; address in Appendix 2), or even suggest that the pupils do a project on the subject of allergy?

My son's school won't let him carry his own asthma inhalers, but makes him go to the school secretary each time he needs to use them. He often doesn't bother. Will this harm him?

It is important that your son takes his asthma medication as prescribed by your doctor. If he needs to take a preventer inhaler at school then, yes, it could be harmful for him to miss this dose, as the control of his asthma is likely to suffer. It is just as worrying if he is not taking his reliever inhaler whenever he needs it. Ideally, this inhaler should be kept with him all the time, so that he has immediate access to it.

Unfortunately, many schools have a policy that all medications needed by children should be locked away. This is usually done from the best of motives – they may be worried that a child will lose their medication, or that it will be stolen, or misused by another child in the class. However, in the case of asthma this is potentially dangerous, and the Department of Health has recommended that all children should have immediate access to their inhalers. The Department for Education and Skills (formerly Department for Education and Employment) document *Managing Medicines in Schools and Early Years Settings* states '**Children with asthma need to have immediate access to their reliever inhalers when they need them.** Pupils who are able to use their inhalers themselves should usually be allowed to carry them with them. If the child is too young or immature to take personal responsibility for their inhaler, staff should make sure that it is stored in a safe but readily accessible place, and clearly marked with the pupil's name. Inhalers should also be available during physical education and sports activities or school trips.'

I suggest that you discuss all this with your son's teachers and try to persuade them to alter their current policy. You could also ask your doctor to write to the school, explaining why it is best that your son has immediate access to his inhalers at all times. You may be able to come to a compromise with the school: perhaps they could keep spare inhalers for your son in case he forgets or loses one. You will also need to persuade your son of the importance of taking his inhalers as prescribed, even if it feels inconvenient for him (I realise that this is easier said than done!).

I have heard that some children have been turned away from nursery schools and playgroups because the staff are not prepared to be responsible for adrenaline injections. Is this true? And what about when the children are older – does this apply to infant and junior schools as well?

Unfortunately you are right. Some private nurseries and playgroups have refused entry to children with severe allergies because, for various reasons, the staff were not prepared to take responsibility for the children's emergency treatment. I think this is very sad, as not only does it stigmatise the affected children but also the staff have missed out on an opportunity to become better informed about increasingly common allergy problems. However, as they are private establishments, they have been acting entirely within their rights.

The situation is different for children in state schools. All children, including those with medical needs, have a right to a full education, and the teachers in these schools should be prepared, within reason, to take responsibility for children's medical needs while they are in school. The DfES document *Managing Medicines in Schools and Early Years Settings* includes details of the responsibilities of education staff, advice on drawing up school policies, and brief information on some medical conditions. Copies can be obtained free from the Department for Education and Skills (address in Appendix 2).

My son has eczema, which at times can be quite severe. I am very concerned because next term his class are to have some intensive swimming instruction. I want him to be able to take part in this, so is there anything I can do to improve his skin beforehand? And is there anything I should do to protect his skin from the effect of the chemicals in the water?

Eczema can pose a number of problems for children when they start to go swimming. Firstly, children can be very shy about the appearance of their skin, often to the extent that they do not want to join in; and, secondly, as you rightly say, there is the concern that the chemicals in the swimming pool water may make eczema worse.

There are indeed steps you can take to try to make the condition of your son's skin better before the start of next term.

- Check with your doctor that the skin preparations you are using are the best ones for your son.

- Be careful to apply his different skin creams as frequently as you are meant to – it is easy to forget!

- Make sure that he has at least one bath a day with plenty of dispersible emollient in the water.

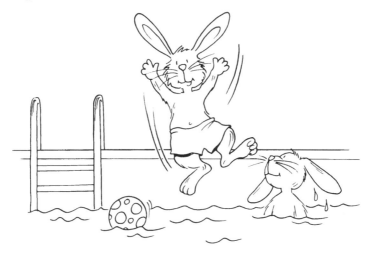

- If you know that there are factors that make his eczema worse, such as certain foods, try to avoid these over the next month or so.

- Make sure that your son wears natural fibres, such as cotton, next to his skin, and avoids clothes made from wool, as these can be very irritating.

- If you know that your son is allergic to the house dust mite, you might consider buying a set of anti-allergy bedding covers.

With any luck, if you follow these suggestions, your son's skin will be in good condition by the time his swimming course starts. However, he will also need to take special care of his skin after each swimming session.

- He should have a shower after swimming, using his soap substitute (normal soap can be very drying).

- He should, if possible, moisturise his skin with his normal emollient (moisturising and softening cream) after his shower, before putting on his clothes.

You may need to enlist his teachers' support, as often the children are rushed to and from the pool and are not given enough time for a shower. Once the teachers appreciate how important this is, I hope they will agree to help.

My daughter has various food allergies and I am worried about how she will cope with meals when she starts school. What can I do to stop her eating the foods that upset her so badly?

The first solution I can offer is to suggest that your daughter has a packed lunch, as then you can avoid the difficulties that school lunches might pose. Most schools have a strict no-sharing policy at lunchtimes. On top of this you should impress on your daughter how important it is for her to eat only the food you have packed for her. If you are still concerned, would one of the teachers be prepared to supervise your daughter while she is eating her meal? All Key Stage I children are now provided with a fruit snack mid-morning. Unless she is allergic to certain fruit, this should not be a problem.

If you want your daughter to have school meals, you will need to ask whether a teacher or dining room supervisor could help her to select appropriate foods. You will need to explain to the member of staff exactly what your daughter is and is not allowed to eat.

This is a problem that should improve with time. As your daughter gets older, it will be increasingly easy for her to understand that there are certain foods she should not eat, and she is also likely to grow out of some of her food allergies.

If she has a serious allergy to one or more foods, it is important that both she and the staff (dining room staff as well as teachers) know what to do if she eats the wrong food by mistake. Chapters 5 and 6, on food allergy and anaphylaxis, will give you more information.

Is it all right to send my son to school when his skin is bad or when he is wheezy? He has both asthma and eczema.

It depends how bad his skin is, and how severe his wheezing. Taking the wheezing first, if he is only slightly wheezy or is getting over a cold but is well in himself, it should be perfectly safe to send him to school. Similarly, if his chest is a little wheezy because he is upset (perhaps for some reason he doesn't want to go to school), then provided that you can make sure he has access to his reliever inhaler throughout the school day, he should be able to go to school. If, however, your son is just developing an attack of asthma, or is wheezy enough for it to interfere with normal everyday tasks, it would be safer to keep him at home until the attack is under control. If you do send him to school, make sure the teachers are able to contact you should his asthma get worse.

If your son's eczema is particularly severe, he may not want to go to school because he may well suffer from teasing or unkind remarks from the other children. He may also feel under the weather because he is not sleeping well. If so, you might want to keep him at home for a few days until his skin has improved. Do arrange to see your son's GP if this happens a lot, as the doctor may be able to make useful changes to your son's treatment and advise you on whether there is anything else you can do, such as using anti-allergy bedding covers (discussed in the section 'House dust mite' in Chapter 9). He may also need a course of antibiotics if his skin is infected. If your son's eczema is relatively mild, there is no reason why he cannot go to school, although it would be helpful if he could take a tube of his emollient (moisturising and softening cream) with him to keep in the classroom to use if his skin becomes itchy.

My 14-year-old son seems to be having more problems with his asthma, and is getting through two reliever inhalers a week. He was fine in the holidays. When I ask him about this he won't talk about it. What could be causing it?

Because he seems to have the problem of increased asthma symptoms only during the school term, we need to think about the possible triggers that might occur at school. It's worth thinking about both environmental and emotional triggers. Although the problem might be caused by dust, mould spores or animal allergens, the fact that he doesn't want to talk about the issue with you signals that it may be an emotional problem. Is he finding his school work difficult? Might he be finding it difficult to organise himself and is becoming overwhelmed by everything he has to do? Or could he be being bullied? Any of these situations could be causing sufficient emotional stress to be affecting his asthma.

It would be worth making an appointment with his class teacher or tutor to ask for their thoughts on the problem. You could also try to get your son to open up to you by asking some sympathetic questions.

If it takes a while to discover the reason for his poor asthma control during the school term, you should make an appointment with your practice asthma clinic so that his treatment can be reviewed.

My daughter is being bullied. Could this be making her eczema worse?

Yes, the upset that bullying causes could be making her eczema worse. Stress is often a factor that is responsible for making allergy problems more severe. In your daughter's case it is affecting her eczema. I hope you find that, once this problem has been tackled, her eczema is less troublesome.

Will my daughter's school make allowances for her hay fever when they mark her GCSEs? The exams are at the time of year when her symptoms are at their very worst.

At present, many GCSE syllabuses contain a major in-course continuous assessment component, so the examinations contribute less weight to the final result than they once did, although this may soon change again. However, exams are still important and there are several steps you can take to ensure that your daughter's hay fever interferes as little as possible with her exam performance.

She should go to see her doctor well before the hay fever season commences, and start taking her recommended treatment several weeks before her symptoms normally appear. This will be much more effective than waiting until after her symptoms have begun. She may need to use a nasal spray as well as taking a non-sedating antihistamine, and if her eyes are affected, she may need eye drops as well (there is more information about all these medications in the section 'Treatment' in Chapter 4).

I hope that treatment along these lines will make sure that her symptoms are minimised. However, it would also be sensible to find out what should happen if her hay fever does affect her badly during her exams, especially as policy varies between examination boards. A letter from her doctor explaining her situation might be needed, for example, or her teacher might need to appeal to the board on her behalf. It might be wise to contact the relevant exam board well in advance of her exams to find out exactly what their attitude would be.

*Is it safe for my son, who has asthma, to go on school trips,
especially ones that involve overnight stays away from home? I
do so want him to lead a normal life, but worry that he might
have an attack and no one would know what to do.*

It is understandable that you worry about your son. However, it is
unlikely that he will be the only child with asthma on the school
trip. Asthma is now so common among children that most teachers
are very well informed about how to avoid attacks and also how to
treat them if they do occur.

To be on the safe side, make sure your son's teachers know that he
has asthma and give them written information about his treatment.
This should include information on what to do if he does have an
attack. You might also like to provide them with some general information about asthma, which you can obtain from Asthma UK
(address in Appendix 2).

*My daughter has severe asthma, and is losing a lot of schooling.
Should she go to a special school?*

Children with asthma should be encouraged to lead as normal a
life as possible, and it is rarely necessary for them to attend special schools. However, if your daughter has asthma that is severe
enough to interfere with her education, it is important that you
know how to make sure that she gets the most out of school and
does not have to miss too many lessons.

The first thing to do is to check that her treatment is as effective as
possible. Arrange to see your GP to discuss both her medication and
her inhaler technique – it may be that something as simple as a
change of inhaler will help improve the control of her asthma (there
is more information about the different types of inhaler in the section
'Treatment' in Chapter 2).

Next I suggest you make an appointment to see your daughter's
class teacher or head teacher to make sure that the school has an
acceptable asthma policy. This should include a commitment to

immediate access to reliever inhalers, staff training on asthma trigger factors, and a plan of action on how to deal with any acute attacks of asthma. If the school does not have such a policy, suggest that they send off for a schools information pack from Asthma UK (address in Appendix 2). They should also have a copy of *Managing Medicines in Schools and Early Years Settings*, which is published by the Department for Education and Skills.

If none of this works and your daughter continues to miss a lot of school, you should contact your local education authority, which will have a person responsible for children with special educational needs. In your daughter's case, having special educational needs is not related to her intelligence but is a reflection of her academic, social and physical needs. It can be a very positive step to be identified as having these special needs, as then something can be done to help.

Every school has a special educational needs co-ordinator (SENCo), who can arrange an individual learning programme for your daughter, talk to your doctor about ways to help her, and show you how you can give her further support. Her progress will be monitored regularly. If she needs even more help, she will be given a detailed assessment, which may, if her school problems are severe, lead to a formal Statement of Special Educational Needs. The Statement sometimes leads to a recommendation for a special school placement, or it may recommend providing extra support to allow your daughter to remain in her current school. The process of obtaining a Statement can take some time and it may require some persistence on your part, so you may want to start finding out about it now. The Department for Education and Skills publishes a booklet called *Special Educational Needs*, a guide for parents that outlines the procedures and explains the jargon used; details of how to obtain a copy are in the website section of Appendix 3.

GOING INTO HOSPITAL

Is it safe for someone with asthma like me to have a general anaesthetic?

Provided that your asthma is under good control, it is almost as safe for you to have a general anaesthetic as any other person. It is important that you continue to take your regular preventer treatment in the month before your operation, and it would be sensible to monitor your asthma using a peak flow meter to ensure that your control is as good as possible (the use of peak flow meters is discussed in the sections 'Diagnosis and assessment' in Chapter 2 and 'Peak expiratory flow testing' in Appendix 1). If your peak flows show that your asthma control is not at its best, see your GP as soon as possible, so that your treatment can be adjusted.

It is very important that you tell your anaesthetist that you have asthma. As well as being a highly trained specialist in giving anaesthetics, an anaesthetist is a fully qualified doctor who will be able to ensure that your treatment continues right up to the time of your operation. The anaesthetist will probably suggest that you receive an extra dose of your reliever treatment with your premedication.

If your asthma is particularly severe, your anaesthetist might feel that it is better for you to have your operation performed under local (or regional) anaesthetic. This is quite common these days, and can be used in a wide range of surgical procedures.

I have been told that you are not allowed to have a general anaesthetic while you have a cold. I am worried that I won't be able to have my operation because my hay fever is like a cold but all the year round. What should I do?

If you are having a routine operation, it is true that an anaesthetist would probably prefer you to be in perfect health before giving you an anaesthetic, and not to have a cold. It is not the blocked nose that the anaesthetist is concerned about, but the effects of the cold virus on the rest of your body. Your hay fever should not pose a problem. Just explain that it is hay fever and not a cold.

It sounds to me, though, as if your hay fever could be better treated. You may need to use a nasal spray as well as taking an anti-histamine: this combination should be able to get rid of most of your symptoms. There is more information about these medications in the section 'Treatment' in Chapter 4.

While I'm in hospital for my operation, will I be allowed to use my inhalers whenever I need to?

The ward nurses would probably prefer that you give them your preventer inhaler for safe keeping. It will then be prescribed for you on your treatment sheet, so you will still be able to use it according to your usual regimen – it will be given to you to use at your normal times.

You should keep your reliever inhaler with you, and use it whenever you need to. However, let the nurses know that you have a reliever inhaler, and tell them whenever you use it. This is because there is a possibility that it might interact with other treatments prescribed for you, and also so that they can keep an eye on how well your asthma is controlled.

Will the hospital be able to provide me with my special diet? I cannot eat eggs or milk.

When you first arrive at the hospital, you will be asked whether you have any special dietary requirements. The hospital kitchen will then be able to provide you with a suitable diet. They are well used to preparing food for people with special dietary needs, and should be able to provide you with everything you need. However, if there is a particular food or drink that you would really miss, take some with you or arrange for your visitors to come well supplied.

The last time I went into hospital, my eczema became much worse. Why was this?

There are two possible reasons why your eczema became worse while you were in hospital. The first is that any hospital admission is a stressful experience, and stress almost always makes eczema worse. The second is that the sheets used on hospital beds are fairly heavy-duty and so can be quite rough, and they are also washed in strong chemical detergents and treated with starch. These chemical treatments are probably what irritated your skin. If you need to go into hospital again, ask if you may provide your own sheets.

I am very allergic to latex rubber, and have to go into hospital for an operation. Will the surgeon's gloves affect me?

There are a number of items used in hospitals that contain latex rubber, including the gloves worn by doctors and nurses during an operation. If you have a severe allergy to latex, it is important that you tell the surgeon and the rest of your health-care team about it. They can then make sure that you are not exposed to items that contain latex. Most hospitals now have a latex-free operating suite, which should remove the risk of latex exposure during the operation.

I have suffered several anaphylactic reactions in the past, and I am very worried about having to go into hospital soon for an operation. What would happen if I had another reaction while under the anaesthetic? Would anyone notice?

I can understand your worry. When you are in hospital you could come into contact with a large number of products that might cause a serious allergic reaction, including anaesthetic drugs, antibiotics, products containing latex and foodstuffs containing peanut. You don't say what causes your anaphylactic reactions, but if you know what it is, it can be avoided. Explain that you have had these reactions and describe what caused them to the nurse who takes your details when you arrive on the ward, the doctors on the team looking after you and your anaesthetist (they will all be wearing name badges and should introduce themselves to you). They can then all make sure that you are not exposed to anything likely to set off a reaction during your stay.

It sounds as if you are worried that there might be other triggers that could set off your anaphylaxis, and that this could happen while you were anaesthetised. This is very unlikely but, if you were to have an allergic reaction during surgery, your anaesthetist (who never leaves you once you are asleep) would know about it very quickly. You are very closely monitored during an operation: any change in your heart rate and blood pressure would be noticed immediately, and treatment swiftly given.

SEX AND PREGNANCY

My wife has a severe peanut allergy, but I adore peanuts. Could I be putting her at any risk if I continue to eat them?

Yes, you could, and there are two ways in which this could happen.

Firstly, if there are peanuts or foods containing peanuts in the house, there is always the possibility that she might accidentally eat something with peanuts in it; for example, if biscuits containing peanuts inadvertently got mixed up with others in the same tin.

Secondly, if her peanut allergy is very severe, it is possible that she could develop an allergic reaction if enough peanut was passed to her from someone who has recently been eating peanuts; for example, by you touching or kissing her after you have been eating them. People have been known to have full-blown anaphylactic reactions after a kiss on the lips from someone who has recently been eating peanuts.

For both these reasons it would make sense for peanuts to be banned from the house, and for you to think very carefully whether you wish to continue to eat them. Your question provides a very good example of the way in which allergies can affect the whole family and not just the immediate sufferer.

Just recently my husband has quite literally been bringing me out in a rash! He has changed the brand of shaving cream and soap that he uses, and my eczema, which had been quite well controlled, now seems much worse. Is it possible that I am reacting to his toiletries?

In someone with extremely sensitive skin it is possible for this to happen, although it is not a common problem. I suggest that you persuade your husband to go back to using the products he used before and see whether, over a period of weeks, your eczema improves. If it does, it is highly likely that your husband's new brand of toiletries were the cause of your problem.

I am allergic to latex, and both condoms and the contraceptive diaphragm give me a severe reaction. Any suggestions?

Most manufacturers now make special hypoallergenic condoms, which are available from most chemist's. One of these is called Avanti, and is made by Durex. Not only are these made from polyurethane rather than latex, they also use a water-based lubricant that does not contain a spermicide, something else that can cause an allergic reaction. Latex-free contraceptive diaphragms made of silicone have recently become available and are prescribable on the NHS. I suggest you try these.

I get wheezy when I make love to my partner. Why is this, and what can I do about it?

There are a number of reasons why making love might make you wheezy. If exercise triggers your asthma, it might be that the physical exertion involved is making you wheezy. Emotion can be a powerful trigger for wheezing as well, so that might be part of your problem. Finally, it might be that your partner is using a perfume, aftershave or other scented cosmetic that is making you wheeze. I suggest that you ask your partner to stop using any strongly perfumed preparations, and that you take two puffs of your reliever inhaler approximately 15 minutes before you make love. This may seem a little premeditated, but it should do the trick.

Will being pregnant make my asthma and other allergies worse?

The effect of pregnancy on asthma and other allergies is rather unpredictable. About one-third of women with asthma who become pregnant find that the pregnancy has no effect on their asthma, and no change is needed in their medication. Another third find that their asthma improves while they are pregnant. The other third experience a slight worsening of their asthma, requiring an increase in their anti-inflammatory treatment. Uncontrolled asthma increases the risk of low-birthweight, premature birth and raised maternal blood pressure (pre-eclampsia), so it is important to work with your doctor to keep your symptoms to a minimum. Because the use of inhaled therapy allows such small doses to be taken, all

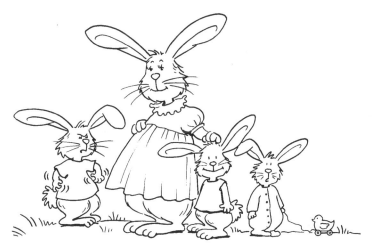

asthma inhalers are perfectly safe to take during pregnancy. If you are using other medications for your other allergy problems, you should check with your doctor that it is safe to continue these during your pregnancy.

There is no way of predicting exactly what will happen to your asthma while you are pregnant. If you feel that your symptoms are becoming worse, it is important that you consult your GP so that your treatment can be adjusted until your symptoms are back under control.

Can I use my usual asthma treatment while I'm pregnant?

Yes, you can. As a general rule, we advise that no drugs be taken by mouth in the first four months of pregnancy, unless absolutely necessary. However, the use of inhaled therapy in asthma allows you to get the maximum benefit with the use of a very small dose. It is important that your asthma is well controlled during pregnancy, to avoid complications such as poor growth of your baby. You may find it helpful to monitor your peak flow recordings until your baby is born, so that you are aware of any deterioration in your asthma control (peak flow recordings and their use are discussed in the sections 'Diagnosis and assessment' in Chapter 2 and 'Peak expiratory flow testing' in Appendix 1).

I am worried that I may have an asthma attack during labour. Is this likely?

No, this is very unlikely. During labour, you produce high levels of two substances, cortisol and adrenaline, both of which are powerful anti-asthma agents. However, it will do no harm to you or your baby to use your reliever inhaler if you feel you need it. Make sure that management of your asthma is included in the birth plan you draw up with your midwife.

Can I use my normal treatments for asthma and hay fever while I'm breast-feeding?

As a general rule, you can continue to take any treatment that is given directly into your lungs or nose by inhaler or spray without causing any problems for your baby. This is because such medications are taken in such small doses that very little, if any, will pass through to your breast milk. However, if you are taking antihistamines or any other types of medication by mouth, these may pass into your breast milk and could have an effect on your baby. It is therefore better to control your hay fever with sprays instead if you possibly can. Remind your doctor that you are breast-feeding so that any prescriptions can be adjusted if necessary.

FINANCE

Are people with allergies entitled to free prescriptions?

This depends on where you live. In Wales, prescriptions are now free but, in England and Scotland, needing medication regularly because you have an allergy does not qualify you for exemption from prescription charges. However, you may be exempt for other reasons – perhaps because of your age, or because you are pregnant, or because you have a low income. A leaflet called *Help with health costs* (booklet HC11) is available from your pharmacist or on-line at the Department of Health website.

If you are not exempt but still need a lot of prescriptions, it may be worth considering pre-payment of your prescription charges by buying a pre-payment certificate (also known as a 'season ticket'), available for either a 4-month or a 12-month period, which allows you an unlimited number of prescriptions. Currently, if you need more than 5 prescriptions in 4 months or more than 14 in 12 months, it will be cheaper for you to buy a pre-payment certificate. To do this, you can:

- complete form FP95, available from most doctors' surgeries, pharmacies and post offices;

- apply on-line to the Prescription Pricing Authority (contact details in Appendix 2);

- buy over the phone on 0845 850 0030.

I am finding the cost of the prescriptions for my severe eczema difficult to afford. I seem to require a large number of different medications, I am not entitled to free prescriptions, and I can't get enough money together at one time to buy a pre-payment certificate. What can I do?

Firstly, I suggest that you tell your doctor that you are having difficulty with the number of different treatments you require, as it may be possible to rationalise your treatment so as to decrease the number of different medications you need. This will not only make it cheaper for you, but could also make it easier for you to use them.

Secondly, there are many preparations (not just for eczema but for other allergies as well) that are cheaper to buy 'over the counter' from your chemist than to obtain on prescription, as the cost is lower than the prescription charge. A considerable number of antihistamine tablets and syrups, nasal allergy sprays and anti-allergy eye drops, most emollients (moisturising and softening creams) and almost all emollient bath additives are cheaper to buy this way. Please don't feel embarrassed to discuss this with your GP, as doctors are well aware of this issue. You could also check with your pharmacist each time you fill a prescription that you are receiving your medications in the most economical way.

If you need a special diet because you have an allergy, can you get any help with the cost?

For infants who are allergic to cow's milk, alternative milks can be prescribed by your GP, and, because the prescription is for a child, it will be free of charge. GPs can also prescribe basic gluten-free foods (bread, flour, pasta, etc.) for people with coeliac disease, although the regulations state that the doctor must be sure of the diagnosis and that the person concerned must be adequately monitored.

No other financial help is available for people with other allergy problems but, whatever the allergy, your modified diet need not be expensive. There are a number of special cookbooks for people with allergies, and more information about them can be obtained from Allergy UK (address in Appendix 2). You might also find the 'free-from' lists available from all the large supermarkets helpful.

MISCELLANEOUS

Should my daughter carry some sort of identification saying that she is allergic to peanuts?

This is a good idea, not just for children but also for adults who are at risk of anaphylaxis or severe asthma attacks, for example. However careful you try to be about avoiding your allergy triggers, accidents can and do happen, and it is vital that any medical emergency team knows about your condition. You can choose between an identity card or a piece of identification jewellery.

Identity cards usually have space to write in your personal details, your doctor's name and address, and some information about your allergy. They may be available from one of the self-help organisations (discussed later in this section) or your doctor may be able to provide you with one. Obviously your daughter would always have to remember to carry it with her and not lose it. Unfortunately, people in the UK are quite reserved and, even in an emergency, will not look through someone's clothes or belongings for such a card, so perhaps the jewellery option is better.

Identification bracelets and necklaces are available from three organisations – Golden Key, MedicAlert and SOS Talisman (their addresses are in Appendix 2). Many people prefer them to identity cards, as they are far more easily seen, more difficult to lose or forget, and by now most of the population knows that they exist and why. Styles vary: on some you have your medical details engraved on the item, whereas others can be unscrewed to reveal a slip of paper containing the relevant information. The back-up provided by the companies also varies, and this may also affect your choice. For example, the MedicAlert Foundation UK (a non-profit-making charity established in 1965) maintains an up-to-date computerised database of details of its members' medical conditions, which they make available via a 24-hour emergency telephone number. Staff, based at the headquarters of the London Ambulance Service, can accept reverse-charge calls from anywhere in the world, in over 100 languages.

Identification jewellery can be quite expensive, but if this is a problem you may be able to find a local voluntary organisation to help you. Several charities, including the Lions Club of Great Britain, support the MedicAlert Foundation and in some cases will help with the cost of joining the scheme. The MedicAlert Foundation or your local library should be able to tell you how to make contact with the Lions if there is a club near you.

When should my son start being responsible for his own treatment? And how can I encourage him to do this?

The answer rather depends on how complicated your son's treatment is, but as a general rule I feel that most children from the age of 5 or 6 should be encouraged to become involved in their treatment in a very simple way; for example, marking off doses taken on a wall chart, or putting together an asthma spacer device. By the age of 7, most children will be able to administer their own medication, but will still need help with remembering to take it.

The age at which a child becomes completely responsible for his or her own treatment will depend on the child – some children can be fully independent by the age of 10, whilst others are still struggling at the age of 17! Many children will be encouraged to take on responsibility for their treatment themselves once they realise that doing so will give them much greater freedom, including the ability to stay overnight with friends, go on school trips, and so on.

The younger you can start your son's involvement with his treatment the better.

I really resent the way that other people treat my allergies as something trivial. They don't seem to realise how difficult everyday things can be when you have these problems, and behave as if they just think I'm fussing about nothing. What can I do? I get miserable enough about my allergies without having to put up with this as well.

It must be very upsetting for you to feel that you do not have a great deal of support from your friends and family. I expect that the reason they behave like this is that they don't know very much about your allergy problems. Part of the difficulty probably lies in the fact that there is such a wide variety of allergy problems, and perhaps your friends mistakenly believe that all such problems are mild. You must also feel angry that your allergies stop you from leading a completely normal life.

The answer is to teach the people around you – your work colleagues as well as your family and friends – about your own allergy problems and how they affect you. You may find some of the educational leaflets from Allergy UK useful (the address is in Appendix 2), or some of the sections of this book may provide you with some of the information they need to know. Getting the facts across will not necessarily be easy, but the more people there are who are well informed about allergies, the easier the lives of those affected will be.

Are there any self-help or support groups for people with allergies?

Yes, there are, and you will find details of a number of them in Appendix 2. The services provided by these organisations vary depending on their size and the amount of funding they receive, but most offer local meetings of support groups, information packs, magazines and telephone helplines, and many also support research. If you cannot find a specific support group for your particular allergy problem, I suggest you contact Allergy UK (address in Appendix 2), which offers help for all people with allergies.

9 | Allergen avoidance

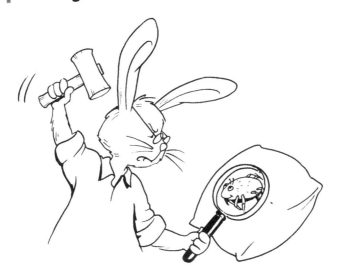

Once you have discovered that an allergy is the cause of your symptoms, it makes sense to do as much as you can to avoid the allergen responsible. In this chapter I describe some practical ways in which you can reduce your exposure to a number of different allergens that commonly trigger different types of allergy problems. More information about these allergens and the conditions they cause may be found in the earlier chapters relating to those particular problems.

Most allergens cannot be avoided completely because they are so widespread. It is still worthwhile avoiding the allergen as much as possible, but you may need to combine this approach with the use of medication. A wide range of medications is available, and they can usually prevent or relieve your symptoms (these treatments have also been discussed in earlier chapters). Remember: the more you can reduce your exposure to the allergen, the more you will be able to reduce your need for medication.

Conventional medical therapy cannot, as yet, provide a cure for allergies, but instead aims to control symptoms by reducing the inflammation that is at the root of all allergy problems, and by making the body less susceptible to the trigger factors that can set off an attack. However, many people dislike taking medications regularly, and find therapies that do not involve drug treatments far more attractive. Chapter 10 looks at complementary therapies, and discusses which of them might be of particular benefit to you.

ALLERGEN AVOIDANCE IN GENERAL

Which are the most troublesome allergens?

The allergens responsible for causing the most symptoms are probably the aero-allergens – that is, those that are carried in the air. The most troublesome aero-allergens are the house dust mite, pollens from grass and trees, and pet allergens, and there are sections on all of these in this chapter. Foodstuffs can also cause problems: although true food allergy (discussed in Chapter 5) is not very common, some foods can act as trigger factors for other allergies, which is why there is a section on them in this chapter.

My daughter has such problems with her allergies that my husband and I would be prepared to move if it would help. Are allergies more common in certain parts of the country, and where would be best for my daughter?

Allergies occur wherever there are allergens, and in the UK that means almost everywhere. However, the amount of allergen in an area can be dependent – at least to some extent – on local environmental, meteorological and geographical features. For example, hay fever can have a definite geographical variation because of differences in the air-borne pattern of pollen distribution; this is why details of the pollen count given in the local media are often more accurate and useful than any national figures.

Allergens are less common at high altitude. Not only are there fewer lush pollen-producing plants and trees, but the house dust mite is less common too, as it thrives in warm humid conditions and dislikes the cool dry air found in mountainous areas. Unfortunately, if you want to take advantage of this you will need to move abroad, because nowhere in the UK is high enough to provide the conditions that deter the house dust mite.

Factors other than allergens also need to be considered. For example, polluted air is not itself an allergen but it can aggravate an existing allergy. Moving from a rural to a built-up area might reduce someone's exposure to a particular plant allergen but the effect of higher pollution levels might then cancel out any benefit gained. Conversely, moving to an area with lower air pollution might remove an aggravating factor but could lead to exposure to a new trigger not previously encountered while living in a large town or city.

As you can see, there is no easy answer to your question, and moving house might not be the answer. However, there are other ways to make life easier for your daughter. Because we spend so much of our lives indoors nowadays, you should pay particular attention to the indoor environment rather than concentrating on outdoor factors. Find out which allergens your daughter is allergic to (your doctor can arrange for her to have various tests of the types described in Appendix 1), and then do whatever you can to make your home, and in particular your daughter's bedroom, as free from these allergens as possible. Details on how to do this can be found under specific allergen headings later in this chapter.

Allergies run in my family. Is there anything that I can do to prevent my children from developing allergies?

This is a very interesting and important question. We currently think that there may well be a number of things that parents can do to reduce the chances of their children developing allergies – asthma in particular – but at the moment we do not have full scientific proof that they work. Studies on a number of potential interventions are ongoing, and we will have to wait for the results before we can recommend these measures. However, I can give you an idea of the areas that are being investigated.

Tobacco smoke

Children of women who smoke become passive smokers of tobacco smoke both before birth (via the placenta) and in early childhood. There is absolutely no question that this increases their chances of developing allergies and asthma. It also increases the risk of other respiratory diseases. Pregnant women, babies and children should *never* be exposed to tobacco smoke.

Diet

Some foods are known to be common triggers for food allergy, and introducing these too early to a baby's diet may increase the likelihood of developing allergy conditions. We think that avoiding cow's milk and hen's eggs in a child's diet until the age of one year may be beneficial.

We know now that some infants show signs of having already developed an allergy by the time they are born, and a number of studies are looking to see whether there is any benefit to the baby if the mother herself avoids certain foods during pregnancy. So far the studies have not shown any positive results, and, for the time being, we recommend that all pregnant women should eat a normal balanced diet.

If, while you are still breast-feeding, your baby is diagnosed as having a food allergy, remember that food allergens such as hen's egg and cow's milk pass across into human breast milk. So, if you continue to breast-feed, you should avoid these foods if you wish to protect your baby from them.

Your baby may be at higher risk of developing a peanut allergy if you, the baby's father or the baby's brothers or sisters have certain allergic conditions such as hay fever, asthma or eczema. If your baby is in this higher-risk group, you may wish to avoid eating peanuts and peanut products when you're pregnant and breast-feeding.

Aero-allergens

Allergens that are light enough to be carried in the air and then inhaled are called *aero-allergens*. If a baby is exposed early in life to aero-allergens such as animal dander (e.g. cat and dog hair), grass pollens and the house dust mite, this may increase the risk of the baby developing allergies. Pollen allergy is more common in infants born just before and during the main pollen season (April to July in the UK) because they are exposed to higher levels of pollen in the first few months of life than those born at other times of the year. We also know that babies born into a household with a cat are at least twice as likely to develop asthma as a baby from a cat-free home.

HOUSE DUST MITE

I have asthma and eczema. I'm also far from being the world's best at housework. Is the house dust mite really so important that I should start making an effort to keep the dust levels down?

For people with house dust mite allergy, the answer is yes, although dusting and vacuuming are only part of the solution. Allergy to house dust mite is the commonest allergy in the UK, affecting 80% of all adults and children with asthma. It also affects people with perennial allergic rhinitis and eczema. However, before you spend time, money and energy trying to eradicate house dust mites from your home, you should discover whether you are in fact allergic to them. If you are not, there is no point in trying to avoid them. Your doctor can arrange for you to be skin-prick tested if there is any doubt about it (skin-prick testing is explained in Appendix 1).

House dust is made up of an enormous number of different things, including fibres from fabrics, lint, food particles, skin scales from humans and from animals, hair, and millions of microscopically small creatures, too small to be seen with the naked eye. The house dust mite (shown in Figure 13) is the most common of these creatures. Its Latin name is *Dermatophagoides pteronyssinus*, and it is

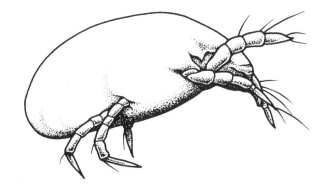

Figure 13 House dust mite, shown 500 times its actual size.

found in almost all of our homes, where it feeds off the skin scales found in house dust.

The number of house dust mites in your home will not vary a great deal throughout the year, although it will tend to be a little higher in autumn and winter. The mites thrive in warm humid conditions, liking best a temperature of around 25°C and a relative humidity of about 80% (conditions found in most centrally heated houses), although they are capable of living in cooler and drier places. The house dust mite is rare in very cold countries and at high altitude, and house dust mite allergy is not a significant factor in the development of asthma, eczema and allergic rhinitis in such places. Because of this, the asthma in children who are allergic to the house dust mite improves when they spend prolonged periods of time at high altitudes.

Assuming that we can't all move to the mountains, how can we reduce the levels of house dust mite in our homes? Firstly, we must look at where the house dust mite lives. The warm humid conditions that the mites like are found in the insides of mattresses, in pillows, in carpets and curtains, and in cuddly toys. Secondly, we must look at what part of the mite causes the problem. It is not actually the mite itself to which we are allergic, but its droppings. This means that even if we were able to kill all of the mites, allergy problems would continue unless we were also able to remove all of the old mite faecal pellets. Thirdly, we must look at how the mite allergen causes problems. It is only when our lungs, or our nasal passages, or our skin comes into contact with the mite allergen that symptoms are produced. If we could put a barrier between us and the allergen, we would be protected from getting symptoms.

The practical steps that you can take to reduce your exposure to the house dust mite allergen are discussed in the remaining answers in this section.

Do I need to buy a new vacuum cleaner?

Not necessarily; it will depend on the model you already own and how effective it is. To reduce house dust mite levels, you really need to use a high-efficiency vacuum cleaner fitted with a special filter that has a pore size of less than 0.3 micrometres. Many ordinary domestic vacuum cleaners are now fitted with this type of filter, and these can be just as effective as the more expensive 'medical' vacuum cleaners. You can find information about each vacuum cleaner model direct from the manufacturers or from the shops selling them. Alternatively, contact Allergy UK (address in Appendix 2), which organises independent tests on many products, including vacuum cleaners, and can provide lists of those which perform to set standards, and which have been awarded the organisation's Seal of Approval.

The bedroom and living room should be vacuumed daily, and preferably when the person with the allergy is not in the room (if you yourself have the allergy, try to find someone to do the vacuuming for you). The machine should be emptied regularly (again you may need to ask someone to do this for you), and the filters replaced according the manufacturer's instructions. As well as vacuuming the carpets, it is worth vacuuming your mattress each time you change the sheets, as, although this won't remove all the mites, it will help to keep the numbers (and the dust) down.

I've been advised that reducing the amount of house dust mite in my bedding will help my eczema. Is this true, and, if so, what should I do?

Yes, if you are allergic to the house dust mite, your eczema may be significantly improved by reducing the levels of house dust mite in your bedroom, particularly in your mattress and bedding. While you are in bed, your skin is in close contact with very high levels of the house dust mite allergen, which can be particularly troublesome if your skin is inflamed or broken.

The following suggestions apply not just to people with eczema, but also to anyone allergic to the house dust mite – after all, we spend more of our lives in the bedroom than in any other single place, and approximately one-third of our lives in bed, so it is an obvious starting place for reducing levels of this allergen. Which of these measures you need to adopt will depend on the severity of your allergy – I suggest you start with the simplest and cheapest first, and only go on to such things as replacing furniture and carpets if it proves to be necessary.

In addition, I suggest that you do not allow any pets in the bedroom (especially not on the bed). Not only can the house dust mite feed on animal dander but also the pets themselves can be major sources of allergens. There is a section 'Pet allergens' later in this chapter.

Vacuuming
Vacuum regularly with a high-efficiency vacuum cleaner fitted with an effective filter (as described in the answer to the previous question). As well as the carpet, vacuum the mattress, the curtains and any soft furnishings such as padded headboards and upholstered chairs.

Bedding
Wash all your bedding (including pillows, duvets and blankets) regularly at as high a temperature as possible (60°C or higher will not

only kill the house dust mites but will also alter the protein structure of the allergen in the droppings and render it non-allergenic). Air it regularly as well, preferably in direct sunlight.

Pillows and duvets

Although it used to be thought that synthetic fillings were better than feather for pillows and duvets used by people allergic to house dust mite, we now know that feather products are in fact preferable. They have been found to contain far fewer mites, and this is due to the much more tightly woven fabric covers used to keep the feathers inside the bedding. These covers have a pore size smaller than the size of the mites, which can't therefore get in. Most feather pillows and duvets can be wet-washed at 40°C.

Barrier covers

Most of the house dust mite in bedrooms comes from mattresses and pillows. The simplest way to tackle these is by enclosing new items in covers that do not allow the house dust mite to get in. Items already

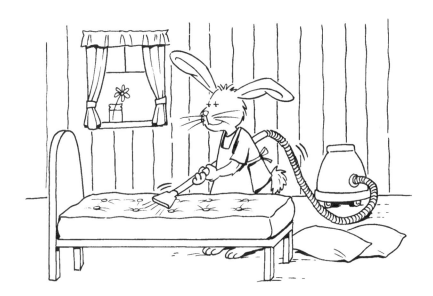

in use can be covered with barrier covers to stop the allergen, found in the mites' faecal droppings, from escaping. They act as a barrier between you and the mites.

I recommend that you ask your doctor's advice before you buy these covers, and that you purchase them only if tests have proved you to be allergic to the house dust mite. They will be a waste of quite a lot of money if you are not allergic to it. If you decide to go for this option, you must use the whole system, which will include a duvet cover as well as mattress and pillow covers.

The cheapest solution is to use plastic mattress and pillow covers. These should be of the type that completely encloses the mattress and pillows, and the zip fastenings should be sealed up with adhesive tape. Plastic sheets are nowhere near as effective, as they do not cover the whole mattress and allow dust to escape from the bottom. The disadvantages of these plastic covers is that they are uncomfortable, as they become quite hot and damp, and they are also noisy when you turn over in bed.

A more expensive but much more comfortable alternative is to use a system of anti-allergy covers made from one of the microporous materials that are 'breathable'. These allow air to circulate, but are so tightly woven that the house dust mite and its droppings cannot escape. Allergy UK (address in Appendix 2) can provide you with information on manufacturers, and will also tell you which of these products have the organisation's seal of approval.

Cuddly toys

Ideally, cuddly toys should not be kept in the bedroom. If toys have to be stored in the bedroom, they should be put in a cupboard or a plastic box with a lid. If a child has a favourite cuddly toy without which he or she cannot sleep, it should be washed once or twice a month at a temperature of at least 60°C. If the toy is not washable, put it in a plastic bag and then place in a freezer for at least six hours (intense cold kills the house dust mite). Then vacuum clean the toy to remove as much of the allergen (which is in the droppings) as possible.

Beds
If possible, avoid sleeping in a bed with a divan base (which itself can be an ideal home for the house dust mite); use one with a slatted base instead. Avoid lower bunk-beds and beds with canopies, as the upper bunk-bed and the canopy can shower dust and mite allergen down onto the person sleeping underneath.

Upholstery and soft furnishings
Padded headboards, upholstered chairs and other soft furnishings provide perfect conditions for the house dust mite, so you may want to consider removing them from the bedroom. If you decide to keep them, they will need regular vacuuming. Curtains should be plain cotton, preferably unlined, and washed regularly. Roller blinds are a good alternative.

Carpets
If you want to have bedroom carpets, those made from synthetic fibres are preferable to those made from wool. Synthetics allow less house dust mite allergen to escape into the air because of a static charge which keeps the mite particles down in the carpet. However, it would be better to have a hardwood, vinyl or lino flooring, as these do not harbour the house dust mite and are easier to clean.

Humidity, ionisers and ventilation
Try to reduce the humidity inside the bedroom by improving ventilation as much as possible. The easiest and cheapest way to do this is to open the windows! If you are allergic to pollen, then, in your pollen season you should open the windows only in the late evening and during the night, when pollen levels are lowest. A dehumidifier will reduce humidity and this may reduce the number of house dust mites in the room.

Currently there is no evidence that ionisers have any beneficial effect on allergy symptoms and at present I wouldn't recommend buying one. I suggest that you try simple measures first, before buying any relatively expensive piece of equipment.

House dust mite sprays

Sprays that kill the house dust mite are called acaracide sprays, and there are a number of them on the market. They are able to penetrate only a few millimetres into furnishings, which means that they are therefore not very effective on bulky items although they might be of use on carpets. I would not recommend that you use these sprays on your bed or bedding, for several reasons: they do not penetrate well into the centre of the mattress and so do not kill all the house dust mites; they do not actually remove house dust mite allergen already in the mattress; and the chemicals they contain can irritate some people's eyes and skin.

What about other rooms in the house apart from the bedrooms?

The next most important room to tackle after the bedroom is probably the living room, but don't forget about any other rooms where you may spend a great deal of your time, such as a home office or a children's playroom. With a little adaptation where necessary, the suggestions I have given for controlling house dust mites in the bedroom apply equally well to the other rooms in the house.

I am considering buying a new home with a heating system that consists of a warm-air unit blowing hot air through ducts from a central heating source to all the rooms. Is this advisable in light of the fact that I am allergic to house dust mite?

This is the worst style of heating you could have! However much you try to keep the house dust mite in your home under control, it is impossible to eradicate it completely. The type of heating you describe will constantly blow the dust containing the house dust mite allergen up into the air where you will breathe it in. It is the levels of mite and mite allergen in the air that matter most, and any device that actively blows air around will lead to increased levels of air-borne dust mite. For this reason, fan heaters and convector heaters are not advisable either. The least troublesome form of heating for people with allergies is gas central heating using radiators provided that the gas boiler is positioned well away from the living and sleeping areas.

POLLENS

Why is pollen such a problem?

Pollens are the male reproductive cells of plants and trees. Pollen grains are very small and very light, so that they can be carried to other plants or trees of the same species and fertilise them. Pollens can be carried by insects or by the wind.

Pollens carried by insects are not usually a problem for people with allergies, as they are heavier and less likely to become air-borne into the air you breathe.

On the other hand, wind pollination is not a very efficient way of fertilisation, so the plants have to produce many millions of pollen grains. These are light and dry so that large quantities can be carried in the air for many miles. This makes these pollens very difficult to avoid, as you will know if you have hay fever or pollen-induced asthma.

I've heard of pollen calendars but I have no idea what they are. How will one help me?

Different plants and trees produce their flowers and their pollens at different times of year, and a pollen calendar shows you approximately when to expect these pollens to be released into the air. An example is shown in Figure 14.

If you have a pollen allergy, the time of year your symptoms occur will depend on the release of the pollen or pollens that are your own particular triggers. Your hay fever treatment will be more effective if begun at least two to four weeks before you expect your symptoms to start. If you want to know what is triggering your hay fever, and can

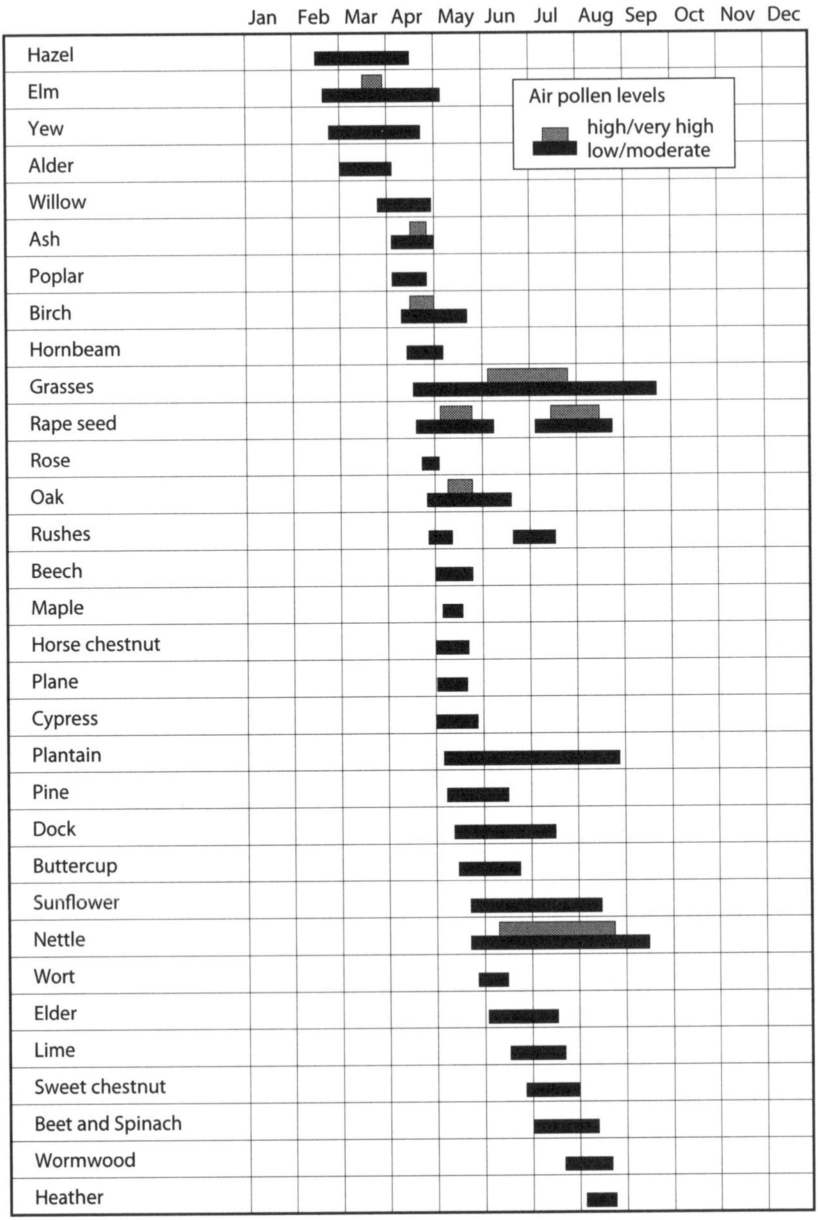

Jan Feb Mar Apr May Jun Jul Aug Sep Oct Nov Dec

Hazel

Elm

Yew

Alder

Willow

Ash

Poplar

Birch

Hornbeam

Grasses

Rape seed

Rose

Oak

Rushes

Beech

Maple

Horse chestnut

Plane

Cypress

Plantain

Pine

Dock

Buttercup

Sunflower

Nettle

Wort

Elder

Lime

Sweet chestnut

Beet and Spinach

Wormwood

Heather

Air pollen levels

high/very high
low/moderate

Figure 14 Pollen calendar

remember when your symptoms start each year, the calendar might help you identify the pollen or pollens responsible. If you know which pollens trigger your allergy, you can use a pollen calendar to warn you when to expect trouble.

A pollen calendar can be a useful guide but you need to remember that unusual weather conditions can advance or delay the pollen season a little. In addition, the pollen count on any particular day will vary according to the weather and atmospheric conditions occurring that day. The pollen count is a measure of the number of pollen grains carried in one cubic metre of air. A count of below 50 is regarded as low, and one over 200 as very high. Unfortunately, if you are allergic to a particular pollen, even a low count can produce severe symptoms.

Everyone else seems to look forward to summer but I dread it because I know that my allergies are going to be at their very worst. What can I do to make my life more bearable during the pollen season?

As I have said before, the most effective way of treating an allergy is to avoid the responsible allergen completely. This is not easy in pollen allergy, unless you spend the whole of your personal pollen season in a place where the plant or plants responsible do not grow, which might be a long way away from home. Not many of us can afford to do this – nor would we want to – and there would always be the chance that you could develop a new allergy to a different pollen. Because it is so hard to avoid pollen, the mainstay of pollen allergy management is to take medications, such as antihistamine nasal sprays and tablets, and other anti-inflammatory treatments as prescribed by your doctor in order to suppress your symptoms.

There are, however, some commonsense measures you can take to reduce your exposure to pollen and so make your summers more enjoyable.

- Spend as little time as possible out of doors on days and at times of day when the pollen count is high, for example in the late afternoon and early evening on fine sunny days.

- Arrange outdoor exercise and sporting activities such as jogging and tennis for those periods of the day when the pollen count is likely to be at its lowest, such as the early morning, late evening or after a rain shower.

- Wearing glasses may protect your eyes from pollen and reduce eye symptoms, so use spectacles instead of contact lenses, and wear sunglasses when you are outside.

- If you have been out of doors when the pollen count was high, change your clothes when you come indoors again, as they will be covered in pollen.

- Keep the doors and windows of your house closed during the day to keep the pollen out.

- If possible, arrange your holiday for the height of your pollen season and go away. Consider taking your holidays in coastal areas where sea breezes keep the air relatively pollen-free, or going abroad to a country where your particular pollen trigger is unlikely to occur.

- Dry your washing indoors (preferably in a tumble-drier) rather than outdoors, as clothes and bedding hung on a washing line can trap pollen grains.

- Avoid mowing the lawn – get someone else to do it. Don't handle newly cut grass.

- Do your gardening on cool, wet or dull days.

- Keep weeds in the garden under control.

- Choose insect-pollinated plants for your garden, as their pollen is less likely to be troublesome.

- Consider buying an air-intake filter for your car or, if you are buying a new car, choose one with a pollen filter already fitted to the ventilation system. These filters are becoming more readily available, and can now be found in smaller cars as well as expensive models.

- Avoid all the other things such as tobacco smoke, dust and traffic fumes, which will make your symptoms worse.

I'm a keen gardener, so how can I reduce my exposure to pollen?

Lots of people ask this question. In response to this, a low-allergen garden was created for Asthma UK and exhibited at the Chelsea Flower Show. Contact Asthma UK at the address in Appendix 2 for further details. You might also find the following suggestions helpful.

- Consult the pollen forecast before going out of doors. A pollen count of 50 or above is likely to bring on your symptoms.

- Do your gardening on cold, wet or dull days. Grass flowers do not open or release their pollen on dull or wet days. In addition, rain washes the pollen out of the atmosphere.

- Do your gardening first thing in the morning when the pollen count is at its lowest. Cool damp mornings – especially when there is dew – will cause the fewest symptoms.

- Don't do your gardening on days when the air quality is poor. Pollution adds greatly to the irritant effects of pollen.

- Try wearing sunglasses while you are out in the garden. These reduce the circulation of air that carries the pollen grains around your eyes. Tight-fitting glasses with large lenses are the best.

- Consider having decorative paving or gravel instead of a lawn. If you decide to have a lawn, get someone else to cut it and dispose of the clippings, and make sure it is cut regularly so that the grasses do not get the chance to flower.

- Choose plants that are insect-pollinated rather than wind-pollinated.

- Don't grow allergen-producing plants such as birch trees, ornamental grasses and members of the daisy family.

- Don't forget that weeds can be just as much a problem as cultivated plants. Control them by regular weeding or, preferably, by mulching or growing ground-cover plants.

A very useful paperback is *Allergy-free Gardening: a revolutionary approach to landscape planning* (details in Appendix 3).

PET ALLERGENS

Which pets cause the most problems for people with allergies?

The most common animal allergy in the UK is to cats, but dogs, horses, rabbits and birds also cause problems. We are a nation of animal lovers, and between 60% and 80% of households have a pet of some kind. When you consider that as many as a third of all atopic people are allergic to animals, you can see that these pets are a major trigger factor. For example, one study has found that exposure to pet allergen may be at least partly responsible for causing over 40% of all childhood asthma in the UK. Infants and small children are particularly at risk of becoming sensitised to pet allergens, and should be protected from contact with furry animals.

If you are allergic to animals, can't you prevent problems by avoiding physical contact with them?

Unfortunately not. Animals produce allergens in a number of different ways: their hair and skin is allergenic, so shed fur and skin scales (dander) are a major source, but the allergens are also present in saliva, urine and faeces (droppings). It is not necessary to handle an animal to come into contact with an allergen – animal allergens can travel in the air, and can also be passed from person to person by way of clothing, and even by sitting on the same chair.

Animal allergens can quickly become widely spread around the home. If you or another member of your family is allergic to animals and you already have a pet, it is not enough to restrict the pet to one room in the hope that the rest of the home will stay allergen-free. No matter where the animal is kept, the allergen will quickly spread, travelling on clothes and shoes, and the allergic person will be exposed to just as much allergen as if the pet was allowed anywhere in the entire home.

In fact, it is not even necessary to own a pet to become sensitised. Animal allergens are so potent that you can encounter enough during your everyday contact with other people to become allergic. For example, even sitting on a bus seat that has been used by an animal owner can bring on some people's symptoms.

Animal allergens can stay around for a long time. If the previous owner of your home or car had a pet, it will take a long period of regular cleaning before every trace of allergen disappears. At least six months of hard work with an efficient vacuum cleaner is needed to clear a house of cat allergens.

How do I know that it really is our dog that is causing the problems? I don't want to have to find him another home unless I really have to.

Many people think that if you are allergic to a pet you will suffer acute attacks of your asthma or eczema or rhinitis when you are in contact with it, and that because of this the allergy will be obvious. In fact, this is rarely the case. Instead, the constant exposure to the allergen keeps your allergy ticking over, making your general condition worse but not producing obvious attacks. If you want to know for sure whether you are allergic to a particular animal (a dog in your case), skin-prick testing or RAST might make this clearer.

Your doctor can arrange for you to have these tests, which are described in Appendix 1.

Have you spent time away from home in a pet-free environment? How were your symptoms then? If they improved after a week or two, it is likely that your dog is a problem. You could consider keeping him outside in a kennel and spring-cleaning the house to remove as much allergen as possible to see whether the improvement can be maintained. You could also try sending your dog away for a 'holiday' (perhaps a friend or relative will take him) to see whether this improves your symptoms. The dog will have to be sent away for quite a while, to give you time to clear most of the allergen from the house, but if your symptoms improve, you will then have your answer.

> *Our son is allergic to our cat but is so distressed at the thought that she might have to go to another home that we have decided to keep her. What can we do to try to keep the allergen level down?*

This is a common problem as, like many other people, your son considers your pet to be a member of your family. The following suggestions may help, but sadly they are unlikely to solve the problem completely.

- Can the cat live outside if you provide her with suitable shelter? Ideally she should not be allowed into the house at all. Your son will need special clothes to wear when grooming her, and you should not bring these into the house either.

- It seems that shampooing a cat every week reduces the amount of allergen it sheds – although this might turn out to be one piece of advice that is easier said than done.

- Use a high-efficiency vacuum cleaner (as described in the earlier section 'House dust mite'), and use it regularly to remove as much of the allergen in the house as possible.

- Try to keep your son's contact with the cat to a minimum. He should change his clothes and wash his hands when he comes into the house after playing with her outside.

I think that it is good for children to have pets but I've read so much about them causing allergies. What pets could we have?

Consider a pet that does not shed allergen, such as fish, or one that is kept in a cage and so is not free to spread allergen around the house, such as a hamster or a gerbil. These have the added advantages of being cheap to keep and not needing long walks! Guinea-pigs and rabbits can be kept outside, and washing your hands after handling them will stop the allergen coming into the house. It is claimed that some particular species of dog and cat are less likely to cause allergic sensitisation – for example, dogs that need clipping and hairless cats – but this is an individual thing (and stroking a hairless cat isn't quite the same . . .).

Alternatively, why not arrange for your child to adopt an animal at your local zoo or wildlife park? This makes an excellent present, need not be expensive, and a wide range of species are available.

FOOD ALLERGENS

Since November 2005 pre-packaged foods sold within the EU are required by law to indicate the presence of 12 major allergens if they are part of the product. These 12 allergens are:

- cow's milk
- eggs
- fish
- crustaceans (shellfish)
- sesame
- cereals that contain gluten

- peanuts

- nuts

- soyabean

- mustard

- celery

- sulphur dioxide and sulphites (more than 10mg/kg or 10mg/litre), expressed as SO_2

By the end of 2007, lupin and molluscs will have been added to this list.

Allergens not on this list will have to be labelled in most cases but there are exceptions. For more information get in touch with the Food Standards Agency (details in Appendix 2).

The legislation applies only to packaged manufactured foods sold in the EU. Exemptions to these laws include foods sold loose, such as bakery or butchery products and delicatessen goods.

Foods of different types seem to be blamed for most things these days – do they cause problems as frequently as some people make out?

Unpleasant reactions to foods are common but not all of them are due to allergy. Personally, I do think it's important to use this term carefully, because if you have a true food allergy, your symptoms may be dangerous, may come on very quickly and can be caused by minute amounts of that food. It is important that people who work with food – for example chefs, waiters and school lunchtime supervisors – take the issue of food allergy seriously, as for some people it can be a life-or-death matter.

We should also treat with respect the other medical problems that can be food-related, such as intolerances, sensitivities and aversions, but in these, the consequences of eating the troublesome food are unlikely to be as sudden or as serious as in food allergy. This is why it is important that we all try to describe food-related conditions accurately. If a chef has numerous requests for dishes free from certain foods each day because of preference or because of mild conditions that the customer labels as food allergy, he is less likely to take the extreme care needed in preparing a dish for someone at risk of food-induced anaphylaxis.

When it comes to other allergic conditions, the role played by foodstuffs in maintaining or provoking symptoms varies between individuals. Certain foodstuffs can provoke wheezing in people with asthma, including:

- peanuts, nuts, sesame, fish, shellfish, dairy products and eggs;

- certain additives, including the yellow dye tartrazine (E102) found in some foods and medicines, the preservative benzoic acid (E210) found in fruit products and soft drinks, and sodium metabisulphite (E220–227) found in wine, home-brewed beer, fizzy drinks, prepared meats and prepared salads.

Some people find that their eczema is made worse by eating certain foodstuffs, and that avoiding these leads to some improvement. This is particularly true in some young babies, whose eczema may respond dramatically to the removal of certain foods from their diet.

Although as many as 50% of young children and 30% of adults with allergic conditions show positive responses to food allergens on skin-prick testing, in most cases these foods do not represent the main cause of their asthma or eczema, and avoiding these foods will not improve their symptoms.

There is now quite a lot of evidence that certain food additives and colourings can cause conditions such as behavioural problems and sleep disorders in children. These effects are not due to allergy but seem to be a chemical sensitivity. It is important not to blame 'allergy' to common foodstuffs for this problem and to needlessly limit the child's choice of foods, their lifestyle and their enjoyment of life by continuing on a special allergy diet.

It is important to exclude foods from the diet *only* if this is appropriate. In this case, 'appropriate' means after talking the matter through with your doctor and confirming, using the correct tests, that a particular food really does affect you in the way you suspect. You can find out more about these diagnostic tests in Appendix 1.

Who can benefit from diets excluding certain foods?

People with true food allergies will avoid provoking their symptoms by excluding from their diet the foods that trigger them. Some people with asthma and eczema may benefit, too. People with food intolerance or food sensitivity – both food-related conditions caused by processes other than allergy – may also need to avoid certain foods. These topics are all discussed in Chapter 5. The more serious condition of food-induced anaphylaxis is discussed in Chapter 6.

Which foods cause the most problems?

In children, the commonest foods causing food allergy are:

- cow's milk
- hen's eggs
- peanut
- wheat
- soy/soya
- tree nuts.

In adults, almost all food allergy is due to the following foods:

- peanuts
- tree nuts
- fish
- shellfish.

If I do need to exclude a food from my diet, how do I go about doing it?

Exclude only one food at a time from your diet, and then only when there is good reason to believe that that food might be the cause of your problem. If no improvement occurs after two weeks, the food should be replaced before another is excluded. Children should not be put on an elimination or exclusion diet of any sort unless you have discussed it first with your doctor. This is because children need the nutrients found in a comprehensive range of food-stuffs to be able to grow well and develop normally.

If you have been found to be allergic to a particular food, you will need to exclude it completely from your diet. This can be difficult, as packaged, pre-prepared and convenience foods sometimes contain some surprising ingredients. You will need to read all food labels very carefully, and develop the knack of spotting all the different names under which particular ingredients can be listed. Remember, too, that manufacturers sometimes change the ingredients they use without any warning, so you must read the packet labels each and every time you buy a food, whether or not you have used it before. I suggest that you consult a dietitian for specialist advice.

Milk-free diets

You must not only avoid drinking milk (whether whole, semi-skimmed or skimmed) but also avoid it in all foodstuffs. This means avoiding foods that contain any of the following:

- milk
- dried milk solids
- milk powder
- milk proteins
- whey
- casein

- rennet casein

- caseinates

- lactose

- lactulose

- lactalbumin

- lactoglobulin

- common foods made from or containing milk, such as cream; butter; cheese; yoghurt; fromage frais; crème fraîche; condensed milk; evaporated milk; most ice creams; most margarines and low-fat spreads including some sunflower spreads; milk chocolate; and desserts such as rice puddings.

Most breads, cakes and biscuits are prepared with milk, as are ready-made or powdered soups and sauces. Breakfast cereals and muesli often contain milk powder. When it comes to drinks, you will need to avoid coffee creamers, malted milk drinks such as Ovaltine, drinking chocolate and 'instant' chocolate-based drinks.

Egg-free diets

You must not only avoid eating eggs (however they are prepared) but also avoid all foodstuffs containing egg in any form. This means avoiding foods that contain any of the following:

- egg

- egg white

- dried egg

- albumen

- some lecithin.

The following foods usually contain egg: custard; puddings; ice creams; chocolate; noodles; pasta; fried rice; cakes; biscuits;

meringues; marzipan; marshmallows; nougat; pancakes; batter puddings such as Yorkshire pudding; sauces; and mayonnaise and salad cream.

Remember that eggs can often be used as glazing on baked goods.

Wheat-free diets

Avoiding wheat means avoiding any of the following:

- wheat

- flour

- starch

- bran

- wheatgerm

- durum wheat

- semolina.

The following foods usually contain wheat: bread; most biscuits (whether sweet or savoury); most cereals; most pasta and noodles; breadcrumbs and foods containing breadcrumbs such as sausages and hot dogs; and any sauces, soups or gravy thickened with flour.

Remember that breads and biscuits made from other grains such as rye and corn usually contain some wheat as well.

Peanut-free diets

If you are allergic to peanuts, you must look out for the following:

- groundnuts

- monkey nuts

- *Arachis hypogaea,* the Latin name for peanut.

The following foods often contain peanut protein: cold-pressed 'gourmet' peanut oil; African, Chinese, Indonesian, Mexican, Thai and Vietnamese dishes; baked goods; sweets; chilli; egg rolls; marzipan and nougat.

Good-quality distilled peanut (groundnut) oil does not contain peanut protein and so is not a risk for people allergic to peanut.

Food labelling laws outside the EU may allow peanut in food to be labelled as nut pieces, artificial nuts and just as flavouring. Because of this, extra care needs to be taken when you are in non-EU countries.

10 | Complementary therapies

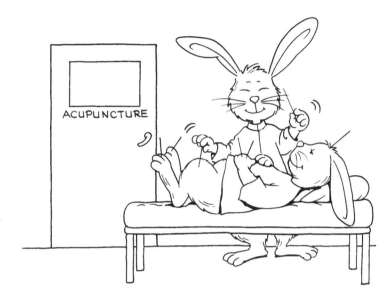

The term 'complementary medicine' describes a broad range of healing therapies that come from world-wide health practices and that are different from the type of medicine used in the UK. They are treatments that their users believe can prevent or treat illness or promote health and well-being. The boundaries between complementary medicine and conventional medicine are not always sharp or fixed.

There is a difference between 'alternative' and 'complementary' therapies. Medicines or therapies that are intended to be used as 'alternatives' – instead of treatments offered by the medical profession – should be viewed very differently from those that are intended to be 'complementary' – those their practitioners intend to be used alongside conventional treatments. No one should stop taking their prescribed allergy treatments without first consulting their doctor, and I suggest that you avoid any 'alternative' practitioners who tell you that their therapies will not work unless you give up your usual medication. Complementary treatments offer their greatest benefits when used hand in hand with conventional treatment, and reputable complementary practitioners recognise this. How to find such reputable practitioners is discussed in the answer to the next question.

Some doctors are rather dismissive of complementary therapies, saying that they have not been proved to work, and therefore discourage their patients from using them. Other doctors take the attitude that these therapies may be a useful aid to relaxation, but that they do little else. Yet others acknowledge that there is an increasing volume of evidence that, in many conditions, several of these complementary treatments are effective. My own opinion is that there is still a great deal that we don't know about the treatment of allergy, and that, provided they do no harm and are used wisely in conjunction with Western medicine, complementary therapies may well benefit many people with allergies.

Complementary therapies are often regarded as low-risk options, but they are not without their dangers. These therapies should be used at the same time as the treatments prescribed by your doctor, which should never be stopped suddenly, as this could be hazardous. In addition, complementary treatments should never be relied upon at the time of an emergency. Acute episodes of asthma and other allergy problems should be managed by fully qualified doctors using conventional treatments. Remember that many complementary therapists have no formal medical training, and might not have the experience or knowledge to diagnose and treat your condition adequately. They may also not be able to recognise certain important complications of your illness. Finally, the treatments used by complementary therapists can themselves be dangerous. Some Chinese herbal medicines have been found to be adulterated with potentially dangerous drugs such as corticosteroids in high doses. The Chinese herbal medicine *Aristolochia* caused kidney failure in several patients and was banned in the UK in 1999. Poor hygiene resulted in 12 patients contracting hepatitis B in 1998 during a treatment called autohaemotherapy. You can avoid problems like this by choosing your therapist carefully. See the next question for some useful tips.

FINDING A GOOD THERAPIST

How can I make sure that I pick a good therapist?

This can be difficult. In the UK there are now over 40,000 complementary therapists (compared with 31,000 GPs) and some are largely unregulated, because registration with a professional body is not compulsory for many complementary therapies. This is very different from the position in the rest of Europe, where registration of practitioners is compulsory in many countries, with only registered health professionals being allowed to practise.

However, there are a number of organisations representing complementary therapy practitioners in the UK: usually each therapy has its own 'governing body' and there are also umbrella organisations trying to improve standards across the whole range of complementary treatments. The BBC Health website has an excellent section on complementary therapies (details in Appendix 2) which gives the contact details of the relevant professional bodies.

There are a number of ways you could find a therapist:

- Ask your doctor if he or she can recommend a therapist. Your GP may know of reputable practitioners in your area, and some health centres now offer some complementary therapies in-house.

- Ask around locally for recommendations. You may find adverts in your local paper, but remember: good practitioners often don't need to advertise.

- Contact the relevant professional organisation. You can find contact details in Appendix 2. This may take a little time, but you will know that the practitioner is appropriately qualified.

Before you start on a course of a complementary therapy, I suggest that you ask the therapist the following questions, and agree to go ahead with it only if you are satisfied with the answers you receive.

- What training have you had?

- What are your qualifications?

- How long have you been practising?

- What experience have you had treating problems like mine?

- Are you registered with a professional organisation?

- What is your attitude to conventional medicine?

- Are you happy for me to continue with my normal treatment?

- Will you liaise with my GP about this treatment?

- What will the treatment involve?

- Is it the best treatment for me?

- Will this treatment help me?

- How many sessions do you recommend?

- What will it cost?

- Is this treatment available on the NHS?

You should be very wary of any therapist who is not happy to answer these questions, or one who claims to be able to cure you.

ACUPUNCTURE AND ACUPRESSURE

I have heard that acupuncture can be useful for people with allergies. Is this true? I would be interested in trying it if I didn't dislike needles so much. Is it as painful as it sounds? Are there any similar treatments that don't use needles?

Acupuncture is a therapy based on traditional Chinese methods, in which fine needles are inserted at specific points of the body to stimulate energy flow and to restore equilibrium in the body. The

Chinese believe that our life-force is based on the interplay of two dynamic forces: yin and yang. In the body, these forces are regulated according to the flow of energy (which they call 'chi') in 14 channels, known as meridians. Most of these meridians connect with a particular inner organ. A blockage in this energy flow results in illness. Diagnosis is not based on patterns of specific symptoms as it is in Western medicine, but on a wider assessment of the individual's mood, character and life situation, as well as a physical examination of the pulses.

Acupuncture may be used for a wide range of reasons, including pain relief, anaesthesia for operations, to help someone give up smoking and for the treatment of asthma. Although in asthma it has produced relaxation of the airways and a temporary increase in peak flow, it has not been shown to have a lasting benefit. Chinese clinics treat people with asthma on a daily basis over very long periods of time: in the UK that would be very expensive and might not offer much advantage over conventional treatments. Acupuncture is also sometimes used in other allergies such as hay fever.

At the beginning of the session, the acupuncturist will make notes on your medical problems, and will examine the pulses on each wrist. Very fine stainless steel needles will then be inserted into your skin at a number of points on your body, the exact number and position depending on the acupuncturist's assessment of the treatment you require. It is important that your therapist uses single-use disposable needles to reduce the risk of infection. The needles will be left in place for between 5 and 30 minutes, and may or may not be connected to a device called an electro-stimulator. The needle insertion is virtually painless, and produces no bleeding. Some people feel drowsy or tired immediately after treatment and should rest before driving or returning to work. Others may feel invigorated.

As you dislike needles so much, you could consider *acupressure*, which uses the same energy system of meridians. Instead of needles, gentle pressure is applied to the acupuncture points. Another alternative is *shiatsu* (the name means 'finger pressure'). This therapy developed at the same time as acupuncture. However, it is more of a general therapy to induce relaxation and well-being rather than one intended to treat specific illnesses.

AROMATHERAPY

As aromatherapy uses oils made from plants, can it be used by people with allergies?

As you say, aromatherapy involves treatment with essential oils, which are aromatic (scented) oils extracted from the roots, flowers or leaves of plants. Most oils are extracted by steam distillation. It is extremely unlikely that anyone would be allergic to these pure essential oils used at the correct dilution. However, some oils are prepared by expression (squeezing) or by maceration (tearing and mashing), and these may contain sufficient quantities of the plant allergen to cause an allergic reaction. Make sure your therapist knows about your allergies, and about the cross-reactivity that occurs between different plants and fruits. More details on this can be found in Chapter 5, on food allergies.

A fully qualified practitioner (you should avoid therapists who are only qualified to give beauty treatments) will ask you about your allergies and will use only oils that will not trigger your symptoms. The oils are chosen so as to balance your body systems. The aromatherapist will make you up your own prescription of oils and give you suggestions on how you can use them at home (in the bath, perhaps, or as an inhalation).

An aromatherapy treatment often involves massage, which in itself can be very relaxing. It may help to relieve any tensions and stresses that might be making your allergies worse.

MASSAGE

What about other types of massage – are they of any use?

If stress triggers your allergy or makes it worse, anything that helps you relax may be useful, and most forms of massage are very relaxing.

One type of massage that is thought to help in asthma (although there is no scientific proof of this) is *reflexology*, a form of foot massage. The foot is divided into zones, which represent the organs of the body. Energy lines or zones are considered to run up and down the feet, connecting the different organs. Massage of the various zones of the foot are claimed to help specific illnesses as well as restoring general well-being. It may work by promoting relaxation – provided that you are not ticklish!

HERBAL MEDICINES

There has been a lot of publicity about people whose eczema has been cured by using Chinese herbs. Is this really effective, and will any other sort of herbal medicine help someone with an allergy?

Herbal medicines have been used for thousands of years, and the medicinal properties of a number of these substances have been confirmed by scientific research. A quarter of all our modern medicines are made from plants that were first used as traditional herbal medicines. These include aspirin and digoxin.

Herbal medicines are made from the leaves, roots, flowers or bark of plants. Although they are regarded as a complementary treatment in the UK, some 60% of the world's population uses no other form of medicine. Side effects are rare but remember: just because it's natural doesn't mean it is safe.

Medical herbalists take a broad or holistic approach to treatment, aiming to use herbal treatments to improve general well-being as well as to reduce specific symptoms. Herbal remedies are used in combinations that are chosen specifically for each individual and his or her problems. To treat an allergy, a herbalist would aim to give you remedies to act on your immune system and so make you react less strongly to your particular triggers, but a reputable practitioner will not claim to be able to cure you of all your symptoms.

The form of Chinese herbal medicine you mention seems to be very effective in certain cases of eczema, and is currently being formally assessed. However, the publicity surrounding it has led to some suspect preparations appearing on the market. Cases of liver damage as a result of treatment with Chinese herbal teas have been reported, and unregulated preparations have occasionally been found to have been spiked with undeclared ingredients such as corticosteroids. Every herbal medicine ingredient should be marked with its supplier's details and should have a batch number to enable its origins to be traced. Be wary of any preparation not marked with these details. Only use the services of a therapist who is registered with one of the recognised professional bodies. As it is very difficult to check the qualifications of therapists trained and registered in countries such as China, I recommend you use a therapist registered with a professional organisation based in an EU country.

Loosely related to the more traditional forms of herbal medicine (and to homeopathy) are the *Bach flower remedies*. In 1933, a doctor called Edward Bach introduced this system of 38 flower remedies in the hope that he had found a simple method of healing. He felt that if he treated his patients' fears and anxieties and relieved them of all negative states of mind, he could free them of illness. These remedies are not commonly used for the treatment of allergies, but are widely available, have no side effects and are unlikely to be harmful. If you do not drink alcohol for any reason, then beware: these preparations contain alcohol.

OSTEOPATHY

I had a bad back and had treatment from an osteopath. To my surprise, my asthma was less of a problem than usual for some time afterwards. Was this just coincidence?

It might have been coincidence, or simply being released from the stress of having a bad (and probably painful) back might have contributed to your improvement. However, some practitioners do feel that osteopathy may be useful in asthma, because it may help to improve chest movement and breathing.

Our framework of bones, muscles, ligaments and tendons supports all of our vital organs. Osteopaths base their treatment on the belief that, when an injury disrupts this framework, the internal organs are affected too. Practitioners take your medical history into account before testing your muscle strength and examining the way you stand and move. Treatment involves massage techniques, stretching and manipulations.

Some osteopaths also practise cranial osteopathy. Although conventional medicine regards the bones that make up the skull as being rigidly fixed together, cranial osteopaths believe that these bones are capable of tiny movements, and that their manipulation may encourage more healthy flow of the cerebo-spinal fluid bathing the surface of the brain, thus facilitating the body's self-healing and self-balancing process. This therapy is not commonly used for allergies.

HOMEOPATHY

I live near a homeopathic hospital and I understand this treatment is available on the NHS. Can you tell me what homeopathic treatment involves, and would it be worth me trying it for my asthma?

Homeopathy is the treatment of like with like. The therapist gives the patient tiny doses of the substance which, in larger doses, would produce the same symptoms that are being treated. Symptoms are seen as the efforts of the body to rid itself of a particular problem, and the remedy attempts to stimulate the body to function more effectively in overcoming the disorder. In addition, remedies can be offered that aim to treat the individual's constitution in a wider sense to resolve long-standing problems. Homeopathy can take some time to show results: initially the symptoms may become worse, and it may be months before a beneficial effect is expected.

The remedies used are natural vegetable or mineral substances that are given in minute quantities. The more dilute the preparation, the more potent it is believed to be. (One of the objections to homeopathy by those who feel it has no genuine effects is that the remedies are so dilute that no trace of the original substance can actually be detected.) Because of this, the remedies are safe, and side effects are rare.

As you say, homeopathy is available through the NHS, but provision is limited. There are five NHS homeopathic hospitals in the UK (in London, Glasgow, Liverpool, Bristol and Tunbridge Wells), and some GPs are also trained in homeopathic medicine, but most practitioners work in private practice.

A number of studies have suggested that homeopathy is effective in hay fever, although none of these has been carried out in the way used to test the efficacy of conventional medicines. As hay fever is a result of the response of the body to plant proteins, it is possible to see how the condition might respond to treatment with related plant extracts. Eczema may also be treated homeopathically. You specifically asked about asthma, but this does not seem to respond as well to homeopathic treatments. Because asthma can be brought on by a large number of triggers in any one person, this is perhaps not surprising.

BREATHING EXERCISES

Are breathing exercises likely to help me cope with my asthma?

The Buteyko technique (named after the Russian professor who developed it) is a system of breathing exercises intended to reduce asthma symptoms by altering the balance of oxygen and carbon dioxide in exhaled air. Those who practise the technique believe that people with asthma 'over-breathe' and, by doing so, lose too much carbon dioxide from their system. However, very little research has been published in medical journals about the Buteyko technique, and this makes its efficacy difficult to assess. It seems that these exercises can make you feel more in control when you are having symptoms, but doesn't improve the underlying condition. (For information about the technique, contact the UK Buteyko Breathing Centre; details in Appendix 2.)

HYPNOSIS

I have eczema. If I was hypnotised, would it help me stop itching all the time?

In some people with eczema (and it sounds as if you may be one of them), itching can be an extremely debilitating symptom and can have a profound effect on the quality of life. When you are hypnotised, you enter a state of very deep relaxation, during which you are more receptive to suggestions of ways of altering behaviour than you would be in a fully conscious state. Although hypnosis is most effective in reinforcing good intentions to change bad habits (e.g. stopping smoking), it may also be beneficial in the management of this type of itching. For other methods of treating eczema, see Chapter 3.

ENZYME POTENTIATED DESENSITISATION

I have read about enzyme potentiated desensitisation (EPD). Is this something that is likely to help my allergy symptoms?

This treatment has been used by alternative therapists for the treatment of hay fever. EPD is a form of desensitisation in which a mixture of allergens (including food allergens and aero-allergens) is combined with an enzyme called beta-glucuronidase and injected in small doses under the skin. Because a mixture of allergens is used, it is said there is no need to determine which allergens you are allergic to before beginning treatment, and the mix used might bear no relation to your allergies.

Because the dose of allergen is smaller than in conventional desensitisation (discussed in the section 'Allergy explained' in Chapter 1), the risk of anaphylaxis (discussed in Chapter 6) is said to be less. However, this treatment is still potentially dangerous and should be performed only where any adverse reactions can be swiftly and properly treated by fully trained, medically qualified personnel. A large and rigorous scientific study has recently shown that EDP is not effective in treating hay fever, and this therapy seems to offer no advantages over more conventional therapies.

11 | The future

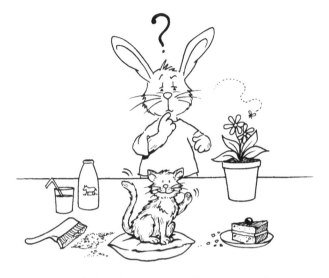

Every year seems to bring important advances in the management and treatment of allergic conditions, but there are still big gaps in our knowledge and, at the moment, we can only treat, not cure, the 18 million people who suffer from these conditions in the UK. However, this may soon change. In 2006, researchers at the Johns Hopkins University in the USA used an experimental DNA-based vaccine in a small number of volunteers to determine whether it could protect them from the symptoms of their ragweed pollen allergic rhinitis. After only six weekly injections, the volunteers showed a 60% reduction in hay fever symptoms compared with those in the control group. The benefit was also seen a year later, although no more vaccinations had been given. The researchers' work is continuing, and they hope their vaccine may be available in as little as three years.

The concept of a vaccination against allergy is very attractive, and other researchers are working on vaccines to protect against the cold virus, which is a potent trigger for asthma in many people, and a vaccine against cat allergy.

Although vaccines could reduce or even eliminate symptoms in those who have already developed allergic disease, it would be an even more exciting prospect to prevent these diseases from developing in the first place.

This is why it is important to learn more about the way in which allergic diseases are inherited, how they develop and how they change over a person's lifetime. If we can discover which genes – the pieces of genetic information on our chromosomes – are responsible for the inheritance of atopy and allergic conditions from our parents, the development of specific drugs that target different aspects of the disease process may be possible.

We already know of some simple measures for the prevention of allergy, the most important of which is never to expose our unborn babies, infants and small children to tobacco smoke. Many other, more complex, measures are being investigated by different groups of scientists and doctors all over the UK. They include changes in the mother's diet during pregnancy and in the infant's diet in the first year of life, targeting the over-use of antibiotics in the population as a whole, and making changes in the home environment during pregnancy and in the early years of life.

Even if research studies give us effective ways of preventing allergic diseases, we still need to find better ways of treating them. There are exciting developments emerging all the time; one of the most promising is the use of monoclonal anti-IgE antibodies in the treatment of asthma and allergic rhinitis. These drugs are now being trialled in food allergy as well. There is new hope for people with severe asthma who don't respond to treatment with corticosteroids; a new finding suggests that vitamin D_3 may make steroids much more effective in these patients. One of the leukotriene receptor antagonists, montelukast, has become available in granule form for infants 6–24 months of age, bringing another oral treatment option for this difficult-to-treat age group. Tacrolimus and pimecrolimus offer us a different way to treat eczema.

In the area of disease management, probably one of the most helpful innovations has been to give patients with asthma more responsibility for their condition and greater freedom to make changes in their treatment regimen according to their symptoms. Patients who have learned to self-manage have improved asthma control and reduced the number of hospital admissions, emergency department visits, unscheduled visits to the GP, and days off work and school.

These new treatments and management strategies, along with the promise of novel treatment and prevention options in the future, combine to provide real hope for the millions of people with allergy in the UK. In the meantime, if you can learn more about what is happening in your body when you develop an allergic reaction or suffer an exacerbation of your allergic condition, you may benefit by being able to turn that knowledge into actions. By avoiding triggers, treating your symptoms earlier and managing your condition more effectively, you will reduce the impact that your condition has on your life. I hope that this book will help you to achieve this.

Glossary

Terms in *italics* are also defined in this Glossary.

action plan *see* self-management plan

adjuvant factors environmental factors such as air pollution and cigarette smoke that can increase an individual's risk of developing an *allergy* problem

adrenal glands important glands in the body which produce a number of hormones (chemical messengers) that are involved in the control of blood pressure and salt and water balance, as well as producing natural *corticosteroids* and *adrenaline*, the hormone involved in the 'fight or flight' response

adrenaline (also called **epinephrine**) a natural hormone (chemical messenger) produced by the *adrenal glands* every time we exercise or are under stress or are scared. It acts on the blood vessels to maintain normal blood pressure and circulation. Adrenaline can also be administered by injection to treat the symptoms of severe allergic reactions

aero-allergen any *allergen* that is light enough to be carried in the air and inhaled; examples include animal *dander* and *pollen*

airway obstruction narrowing or blockage of the passages that carry air to and from the lungs

allergen a normally harmless substance that can trigger an allergic reaction; once an *allergy* has developed, even a tiny amount of the allergen can lead to a reaction and cause allergic symptoms

allergen immunotherapy another name for *desensitisation*

allergic rhinitis inflammation of the lining of the nasal air passages caused by an *allergy*; depending on the *allergen* involved, it may be seasonal (*hay fever*) or occur all year round (*perennial allergic rhinitis*)

allergic sensitisers another name for *sensitisers*

allergy an abnormal or inappropriate reaction of your body's *immune system* to a substance that would normally be harmless (an *allergen*)

anaphylaxis a sudden severe allergic response to an *allergen*, a potentially life-threatening reaction that involves the whole body. If untreated, it can lead to dizziness, shortness of breath, *wheezing*, palpitations, swelling and obstruction of the upper airway, a serious drop in blood pressure and collapse. Emergency treatment is with *adrenaline* injections

angioedema swelling of the deep layers of the skin (the dermis) as a result of an allergic reaction; the parts of the body most commonly affected are the face and lips

antibodies or **immunoglobulins** produced by the *immune system* in response to a foreign substance, antibodies circulate in the blood and help to fight infection. They act as the immune system's memory, recognising harmful attackers such as bacteria and viruses the body had encountered before, and assisting in their destruction

antihistamines drugs that block the action of *histamine*; they are used to treat *allergy* problems such as *hay fever* and insect stings

anti-inflammatory drugs drugs that act against *inflammation*. Many diseases or conditions of the body – from *asthma* to arthritis to bowel disease – are characterised by inflammation. Anti-inflammatory drugs reduce this inflammation and help the body to keep functioning as normal

asthma a condition in which *inflammation* of the airways and twitchiness of the airway wall muscles make it difficult to move air in and out of the lungs, and causes the symptoms of *wheezing*, coughing and tightness of the chest

atopic dermatitis another name for *eczema*

atopy a tendency to develop allergic disorders such as *asthma*, *hay fever* and *eczema*. This tendency is inherited genetically from your parents

biopsy the removal of a small piece of body tissue, which is then examined under a microscope for diagnostic purposes

brand name or **trade name** most drugs have at least two names: the brand or trade name is the name given to the drug by its manufacturer, and is usually written with a capital first letter. The other name is the *generic* (or pharmaceutical) *name*. Any one drug can have several brand names but only one generic name

bronchoconstriction narrowing of the airways due to tightening of the muscles in the airway walls

bronchodilators drugs used in treating *asthma* that relax the muscles of the airway walls and so open up (dilate) the airways. They can be taken by *inhaler* or by mouth. The medical term for *relievers*

challenge tests or **provocation tests** sometimes the only way to confirm an *allergy* is deliberately to provoke the symptoms it causes, using a challenge test. A small amount of a substance thought to be responsible for an allergic reaction is given in an appropriate way (e.g. by mouth for a food, by inhalation for an *aero-allergen*) and the resulting symptoms recorded. Challenge tests can also be used to demonstrate that a particular allergen is **not** responsible for symptoms. The tests may be *single blind* or *double blind*

chromosome one of 46 pieces of genetic material present in all cells of the body. Each chromosome consists of a large number of *genes* carrying information inherited from our parents

coeliac disease a life-long inflammatory disorder of the small intestine caused by an *intolerance* to *gluten*

co-factors additional factors that, when combined with an *allergen*, can make an allergy worse. They act as additional *triggers*

complementary therapies non-medical treatments that may be used in addition to conventional medical treatments. Popular complementary therapies include acupuncture, aromatherapy, homeopathy and osteopathy

conjunctivitis *inflammation* of the conjunctiva, which is a delicate membrane that lines the eyelids and covers the eyeball. The symptoms of conjunctivitis are itching, watering, discharge and redness of the eyes

corticosteroids a group of chemicals produced naturally in the body by the *adrenal glands*, which are vital for the body's own defences against infection and stress. Corticosteroids can also be manufactured synthetically. Used as *anti-inflammatory drugs*, they are powerful agents in the treatment of disorders that produce *inflammation*, such as *asthma*, *eczema*, *hay fever*, *angioedema* and *anaphylaxis*

cromoglicate or **disodium cromoglicate** an *anti-inflammatory drug* used in the treatment of *asthma* and *hay fever*

Crosby capsule a small (less than 1 cm long) device used for taking a *biopsy* of the small intestine in order to diagnose *coeliac disease*

dander tiny flakes of skin, covered in dry sweat and saliva, found on an animal, something like dandruff in humans. Dander carries the animal's characteristic allergen in the air, so is an *aero-allergen*

decongestants treatments that reduce swelling and congestion. Nasal decongestants are sprays or drops that relieve nasal congestion; however, because they can cause thinning and drying of the lining of the nose, they should not be used on a regular basis

denature the permanent alteration of a protein when it is heated (or cooked), which may make it less allergenic

depigmentation loss of the skin's natural colour (pigment is the substance that gives skin its colour)

dermatitis an inflammatory reaction affecting the skin. In this book, the term used as a shorthand term for allergic contact dermatitis, caused by contact between the skin and an *allergen*. Contact may occur in a variety of ways, for example by touching the substance, swallowing a drug or being exposed to a chemical at work

dermatologist a doctor who specialises in the treatment of problems and disorders of the skin

desensitisation or **immunotherapy** or **allergen immunotherapy** or **hyposensitisation** a form of treatment for *allergy* in which a series of injections of very small but increasing quantities of an *allergen* are given over several months. These are given in an attempt to reduce or even eliminate symptoms of the specific allergy by building up the *immune system*'s tolerance to the allergen. Because this treatment is potentially dangerous, it is available only in certain circumstances in specialist centres. *See also* sublingual immunotherapy

dietitian a person trained in nutrition who can give advice about all aspects of food and diet

disodium cromoglicate *see* cromoglicate

dispersible something that will mix in; e.g. a dispersible bath oil will mix in with the bath water rather than just settling on the top of it

diurnal variation the change seen between one time of day and another (usually 12 hours later), in a function such as *peak expiratory flow*. In practical terms, this means the difference between readings taken first thing in the morning (which tend to be lower) and those taken in the evening (which tend to be higher)

double blind describes a test (e.g. a *challenge test*) during which neither the doctor administering the test nor the person taking it knows whether the actual substance or a dummy substance is being given at any particular time. This means that the results cannot be biased by the expectations of either party. Someone who is not involved in the testing process keeps all the records

eczema or **atopic dermatitis** a chronic (long-lasting) inflammatory condition of the skin. In mild cases the skin is dry and scaly, but it can become red, blistered and weepy if the eczema is severe. The inflamed skin can also become infected. In eczema, the *inflammation* makes the skin very itchy

elimination diet or **exclusion diet** a method of confirming that a food is responsible for an allergic reaction by removing it from and then later returning it to the diet and symptoms are recorded in a *symptom diary*. Often different foodstuffs are tried one by one, to discover which food is causing the problem

emollient a substance, usually in the form of a cream or ointment, that moisturises, softens or soothes the skin

enteropathy any disease of the intestine (bowel)

epinephrine *see* adrenaline

erythema redness of the skin, often caused by *inflammation*

exclusion diet another name for an *elimination diet*

extrinsic/intrinsic asthma an attempt to classify *asthma* either as being triggered by an external factor such as an *allergen* (i.e. extrinsic) or as not being associated with any obvious allergic *trigger* (i.e. intrinsic). These terms are becoming less commonly used

food diary a type of *symptom diary* that lists each and every food you have eaten alongside any symptoms you have had

gastroscope a flexible tube-like viewing instrument that uses fibreoptic technology to view the interior of the stomach and upper intestine

generic name most drugs have at least two names: the generic name is the true or scientific name (usually written with a small first letter), and normally applies to all the versions of that drug, regardless of the manufacturer. The other name is the *brand* (or trade) *name*

genes the 'units' of heredity that determine the characteristics we inherit from our parents

gluten a protein found in wheat, rye, barley and to some extent oats, which provokes an inflammatory response in people with *coeliac disease*

hay fever or **seasonal allergic rhinitis** allergic reaction to a seasonal plant *pollen* or mould spore; an *aero-allergen*. Typical hay fever symptoms include a runny or stuffed-up nose, sneezing and watery eyes. They occur only during the part of the year when the pollens to which someone is allergic are being produced

hereditary the process of genetically transmitting characteristics from parent to offspring

histamine a chemical released by the cells of the body during an allergic reaction. Histamine causes *inflammation* and the symptoms of *allergy*

hives another name for *urticaria*

house dust mites microscopically tiny creatures, too small to be seen with the naked eye, which live in soft furnishings, carpets and bedding in all our homes, and which live off the human skin scales that we shed all the time. Their faecal particles (droppings) contain a potent *allergen*

Hymenoptera the Order of insects that includes wasps and bees, which are the insects whose stings are most often responsible for allergic reactions

hyper-immunoglobulin E syndrome or **hyper-IgE syndrome** a rare condition in which vast quantities of *IgE* are made by the *immune system*. This leads to an exaggerated tendency towards allergic disorders, particularly *asthma* and *eczema*

hypoallergenic 'hypo' means 'less than' or 'lower in', so products described as hypoallergenic are lower in *allergens* than the conventional formulations. They may well be free from the commonest substances known to cause allergic reactions, but this does not mean that they are completely allergen-free

hyposensitisation another name for *desensitisation*

idiopathic a description that means 'of unknown cause'. When applied to a disease or a disorder, it means that the cause of the problem is either not known or has not yet been identified, for example idiopathic *anaphylaxis*

IgE or **immunoglobulin E** the allergy *antibody*. People with allergies readily produce large amounts of IgE

immune system the network within the body that protects us from outside 'attackers' including viruses, bacteria and parasites, and from other conditions such as cancer

immunoglobulins another name for *antibodies*

immunotherapy another name for *desensitisation*

inflammation the body's response to injury, infection or disease. Inflammation is a reaction involving swelling, redness, tenderness or pain, itching and increased watery secretions. Generally, its purpose is to protect the body against the spread of injury or infection. In some conditions, such as *asthma* and *eczema*, the inflammation is inappropriate (because the *allergen* poses no real threat) and becomes chronic (long-lasting), tending to damage the body rather than protect it

inhalers devices used to deliver drugs so that they can be breathed into the lungs instead of being swallowed or given by injection. Inhalers are the most efficient way of giving *asthma* medications: the drugs work more quickly when inhaled (because they are delivered directly to the lungs where they are most needed) and smaller amounts can therefore be used to produce the same results

intervention any change made in an attempt to alter a disease process, such as reducing levels of *house dust mite* or starting an *elimination diet*

intolerance an inability of the body to handle a substance adequately, resulting in unpleasant symptoms. For example, people who have lactose intolerance cannot digest milk properly because they lack the body chemical (an enzyme called lactase) needed to break down lactose (the sugar in the milk). Drinking milk may give them crampy abdominal pain and diarrhoea. These symptoms are not allergic in nature, and will not occur if only tiny quantities of milk are drunk

intradermal tests diagnostic tests used to identify to which *allergens* someone is allergic by injecting small amounts of diluted allergen extract under the skin. Now rarely used in the UK

intrinsic asthma *see* extrinsic/intrinsic asthma

latent temporarily concealed; i.e. there are no symptoms but the disease or disorder is still present

latex form of rubber used in the manufacture of protective gloves and similar products

legume the pea and bean Family of foods. The Family includes soya bean and peanut, both of which are common causes of *allergy*

metered dose inhaler the most common form of *inhaler* used to deliver *asthma* treatments

monoclonal antibody an *antibody* produced by a single clone of cells grown in culture

multiple RAST a form of *RAST*, which can test for several *allergens* at once

nebulisers devices that convert liquid medication into a fine mist, which can then be inhaled. Nebulisers usually run on compressed air produced by an electric compressor

nedocromil an *anti-inflammatory drug* used in the treatment of *asthma* and *hay fever*

nettle rash another name for *urticaria*

occupational allergy or **workplace allergy** an *allergy* that is the direct result of contact with or exposure to an *allergen* found in the work environment

over-the-counter medications or **OTC medications** treatments that can be bought from pharmacists without a doctor's prescription

passive smoking breathing in smoke from another person's cigarette, cigar or pipe

patch tests diagnostic tests used to identify to which *allergens* someone is allergic; particularly useful for *dermatitis*. A small quantity of the substance to be tested is applied directly to the skin, covered, and left in place for 48 hours

peak expiratory flow or **peak flow** a measure of how hard you can blow; i.e. the rate at which you can expel air from your lungs. It is used to show how well your lungs are functioning, and to detect changes in lung function

peak flow meter a small hand-held device that measures *peak expiratory flow*

perennial allergic rhinitis allergic reaction to an *aero-allergen* that is present throughout the year; e.g. the *house dust mite* or animal *dander*. Symptoms are similar to those of *hay fever* but occur all the year round

pollen small grains produced by plants as an essential part of the reproductive process. The pollen grains are the male seeds, which are light enough to be spread through the air or by insects to other plants in order to pollinate (fertilise) them. Although they are too small to be seen by the naked eye, they are potent *allergens*, and trigger *hay fever*

pollen calendar different plants and trees produce their flowers and their *pollens* at different times of the year, and a pollen calendar shows approximately when to expect these pollens to be released into the air

pollen count the number of *pollen* grains found in a cubic metre of air. A count of below 50 is regarded as low, and one of over 200 as very high. *Hay fever* symptoms are usually worse when the count is high

predisposition susceptibility to a specific disease or disorder

prevalence a measure of the number of people in the population with a particular medical condition at any one time. For example, if we were to say that the current prevalence of *asthma* in the UK is 10%, we would mean that 10% (1 in 10) of the population currently has asthma

preventers drugs that are taken to prevent the symptoms of *asthma* from occurring, rather than to relieve them when they do occur. Preventers do not work immediately, but instead act over a period of time to reduce *inflammation* and stabilise the asthma. The most important preventers are the inhaled *corticosteroids*

provocation tests another name for *challenge tests*

psychosomatic relating to the influence that the mind can have on physical well-being

PUVA abbreviation for 'psoralen plus ultraviolet A', a treatment used for a number of skin conditions, including *eczema* and psoriasis. Psoralen is a plant extract that is taken by mouth. Two hours after taking it, the person being treated lies or sits under a machine rather like a sun lamp, which produces the type of light called ultraviolet A

RAST or **radioallergosorbent test** a blood test that measures the amount of specific *IgE* your *immune system* has produced against an *allergen*. For example, if you have *asthma*, it can confirm that you have *antibodies* against the *house dust mite*. The total amount of IgE in the blood-stream is usually measured at the same time, so that the amount of any specific IgE that is found can be put into perspective

relievers drugs that are used to provide quick and effective relief from the symptoms of *asthma*. They should be used only when symptoms occur and before exercise. The medical name for relievers is *bronchodilators*

rhinitis *inflammation* of the lining of the nasal air passages. *Hay fever* (or *seasonal allergic rhinitis*) and *perennial allergic rhinitis* are the allergic forms of rhinitis

rhinitis medicamentosa chronic *rhinitis* caused by the overuse of nasal *decongestants*

seasonal allergic rhinitis another name for *hay fever*

self-management plan a formal written action plan, drawn up and agreed by you and your doctor, that allows you to take more responsibility for and control of your own treatment. It sets out the circumstances in which you can take action (e.g. altering the dose of your medication) without first having to check with your doctor. Self-management plans often lead to an improvement in the control of an allergic disorder

sensitisers or **allergic sensitisers** substances that can cause *allergies*. This term is used for substances encountered in the work environment that can cause *occupational allergies*

sensitivity a reaction to a substance that is an exaggeration of a normal *side effect* produced by that substance. For example, if salbutamol (a *reliever* drug used in treating *asthma*) is given in a high enough dose, most people will develop shakiness and feel 'revved up'. People who develop these effects at a normal dose are said to be sensitive to the drug, but they are not allergic to it

side effect almost all drugs affect the body in ways beyond their intended actions. These unwanted 'extra' effects are called side effects. They vary in their severity from person to person, and often disappear when the body becomes used to a particular drug

single blind describes a test (e.g. a *challenge test*) in which only the doctor administering the test knows whether a real or a dummy substance is being given. The person taking the test does not know which substance is which, so their ideas about what causes their symptoms cannot bias the results

sinuses the bones of the face are not solid, but have hollow spaces within them. These spaces are the sinuses, which are joined to the air passages of the nose by small openings

sinusitis infection or *inflammation* of the *sinuses*. The openings of the sinuses become blocked and their drainage system disturbed. Once blocked, the pressure in the sinuses can increase because of the build-up of secretions, leading to pain which can be felt above the eyebrows, either side of the nose or in the upper teeth

skin-prick test a diagnostic test used to identify which *allergens* someone is allergic to. A drop of a liquid preparation of the concentrated allergen is applied to the skin on the back or on the inside of the forearm, and the skin is then pricked through the droplet. The response is measured after 10–15 minutes. The procedure is painless, gives rapid results, and is probably the most commonly used and the most informative allergy test

standardised an established measure or model to which other similar things should be compared and to which they should conform. For example, the results of a standardised test performed in one hospital should mean the same as the results of the same test carried out in a different hospital

steroids in this book, a short form for *corticosteroids*

sublingual immunotherapy a new form of *immunotherapy* in which a pill is dissolved under the tongue once a day for eight weeks before the pollen season starts. This method has cut symptoms by up to 40% in over 80% of people who have used it, and it is much safer than conventional immunotherapy

symptom diary a record of your symptoms and the factors thought to be causing them. People who have an allergic problem are often completely well on the day on which they see their doctor, so it is therefore very useful for a doctor to see a detailed record of how serious the problem is, what form it takes and what might be provoking it

trade name another name for a *brand name*

triggers or **trigger factors** popular name for anything that may bring on allergic symptoms or make them worse. For example, triggers for *asthma* include exercise, emotion, changes in air temperature and air pollution

urticaria or **nettle rash** or **hives** swelling of the superficial layers of the skin, usually as a result of an allergic reaction. The characteristic itchy lumps (called *weals* or hives) last for only a few hours

weal a bump in the skin produced as a response to an *allergen*

wheeze or **wheezing** a high-pitched noise produced when breathing out. It comes from the chest and not the throat

workplace allergy another name for an *occupational allergy*

Appendix 1 – Diagnosing your allergies

If you have symptoms that you think may be due to an allergy, it is important that your condition is accurately diagnosed so that, with the help of your doctor, you can draw up an appropriate management plan. If allergy is responsible, you will find details of the treatments available in the individual chapters on the different allergic conditions (Chapters 2–7). If the problem is not the result of an allergy, then, with this knowledge, you can take appropriate steps to find the real cause of your symptoms.

In this appendix I give you a description of each of the common allergy tests, including details of what you will feel and whether they are uncomfortable. I suggest when each test may be needed, point out any special instructions relating to the tests, and discuss their individual strengths and weaknesses in making a diagnosis of allergy. I hope this information will help you to understand why your doctor has chosen one test rather than another. I also briefly describe a number of tests sometimes used by practitioners of complementary therapies, although few of these are felt to have a place in the diagnosis of allergy.

WHY TEST?

If you have had an allergic reaction and its cause is uncertain or unknown, you will need to undergo one or more of the tests described here. Even if you know the cause of your allergic reaction, you may still need to have the diagnosis confirmed by some form of allergy testing, particularly if you have had a severe allergic reaction, or have multiple allergies, or if your doctor is considering any form of treatment that is going to be long-lasting, difficult, time-consuming or expensive. If you are going to help with the evaluation of a new treatment, you will certainly need to have your allergy confirmed by formal testing. If there is any confusion as to whether your problem is caused by a true allergy (that is, one involving the production of the allergy antibody IgE, as discussed in the section 'Allergy explained' in Chapter 1) or whether some other process is involved, allergy testing can clear up this doubt. Finally, if having an allergy has any legal implications for you (for example, if you might be eligible for compensation), the diagnosis must be confirmed by appropriate tests.

As many as a third of the population of the UK currently experience an allergic problem of some kind. Because these problems are now so common, allergy testing is being used more often and is becoming increasingly sophisticated. However, there is no point in doing allergy tests if either you or your doctor is going to be unwilling to take action based on the results. If a true allergy is diagnosed, you may benefit not only from medications aimed at treating the allergic reaction once it has happened but also from taking preventative action, both in the form of drugs and in the form of allergen avoidance.

CHOOSING THE MOST SUITABLE TEST

Different allergies are more common at different ages, and so the type of allergy test you will be offered by your doctor depends, to some extent, on your age. Food allergies are more common in infancy and early childhood, whereas problems caused by allergens in the air become more common after the age of 5 years. Allergies to insect stings usually start in adulthood, and can be particularly troublesome in the elderly.

When we undergo medical tests, we want those tests to be reliable, but what exactly does that mean? Every test used in the diagnosis of allergies should be:

- relevant – there is no point in doing skin-prick testing or patch testing unless you include the likely culprits;

- standardised – so that the result of a test done in one hospital means the same as that done in a different hospital;

- repeatable – so that the results on one occasion can be compared with the results of the same test on a different occasion;

- specific – so that the test is positive only in people who have that allergy; and

- sensitive – so that the test is negative only in people who do not have the problem.

This is a lot to ask of any test, and it is impossible for any one test to score 100% on all of these points. Every test has its advantages and its disadvantages, and this is why specialist knowledge is necessary to make sure that the right test is chosen for you.

Before you get as far as any tests, the most useful information available to your doctor will come from your medical history – the account that you give of your allergic reaction and your answers to a large number of questions, including the following:

- your general status (age, job, and so on);

- the details of your current medical problems;

- any illnesses you have had in the past;

- whether there are other members of your family with allergic problems;

- how often you are exposed to allergens and to other factors that can make allergy problems worse (e.g. cigarette smoke, air pollution and certain drugs).

All of these details must be taken into account when choosing and assessing the result of any allergy test. Although some of these tests are available in certain GP surgeries, if your allergy is particularly troublesome or if you have had even one severe allergic reaction, you should be referred to an allergy specialist.

SKIN-PRICK TESTING

Description

This is probably the most commonly used allergy test. It is performed on the skin of your inner forearm (as shown in Figure 15) or on your back, and an adult can be tested to up to 25 allergens at any one time. A drop of the standardised allergen extract is placed on your skin, which is pricked through the drop using a lancet (a small, sharp prong just 1 mm long). This may feel mildly uncomfortable but is not painful. After 15 minutes, the test site is examined. A positive result consists of a weal (a pale bump), which may be itchy and surrounded by a red area or flare. The size of the weal is measured, and any weal greater than 2 mm in size is regarded as a positive response.

Two additional substances will always be included in this form of testing: a positive and a negative *control*. The positive control solution

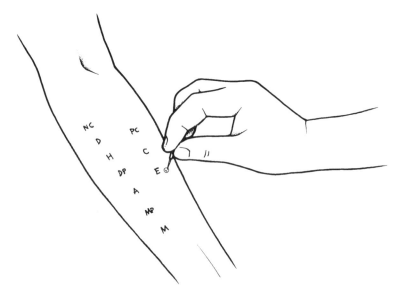

Figure 15 Skin-prick testing on the skin of the inner forearm

contains histamine, to which everyone should react. Failure to do so can result from treatment with certain medicines (including antihistamines, corticosteroids and certain antidepressant drugs) and will alert the tester to the fact that the results of testing will be unreliable. The negative control is made from a saline solution, to which no one should react. A positive reaction to this negative control shows that the skin is, for some reason, extremely sensitive, and once again indicates that testing will not be reliable.

Skin-prick testing is a painless procedure that is well tolerated even by small infants. Positive reactions may be somewhat itchy, but this will subside within an hour.

Skin-prick testing is a very sensitive diagnostic tool, and not everyone who has a positive test has symptoms of an allergy. A positive reaction may be highlighting a hidden or latent allergy that is not currently causing you problems but which might show up later on in your life.

If you do not develop a reaction to an allergen but the positive control solution has produced a weal, you can be fairly sure that you are not allergic to that allergen.

Indications
Skin-prick testing is usually the first test recommended when an allergy is suspected.

Special instructions
Tell the person doing the skin-prick testing if you are on any medication. If it is safe to do so, treatment with antihistamines, corticosteroids or tricyclic antidepressants should be stopped for an appropriate time (up to two weeks) before the test is carried out. However, these medications should be stopped *only* on your doctor's instructions.

Advantages
This is a simple, quick and inexpensive form of testing, which can be performed to a very wide range of different allergens. It can give use-

ful information in all forms of allergy, and provides results within 15 minutes.

Disadvantages
Skin-prick testing is unreliable in the very young and the elderly. It cannot be performed if you are taking certain medications (listed a little earlier in this section) or in people with severe eczema. Generally extremely safe, skin-prick testing may provoke a severe allergic reaction in people who have previously experienced anaphylaxis (discussed in Chapter 6), although this is extremely rare.

INTRADERMAL TESTING

Description
'Intradermal' literally means 'within the skin', from the Latin word *intra* meaning 'within' and the Greek word *derma* meaning 'skin'. In this test a small amount of a diluted allergen extract is injected beneath the surface of your skin using a needle and syringe. A reaction is usually apparent within 10–20 minutes, and takes the form of swelling, itching and a raised weal (a pale bump).

This form of testing is now rarely used in the UK; not only does it give inaccurate results (using a high concentration of allergen can falsely indicate allergy where none exists) but also it can be dangerous, with a higher risk of anaphylactic reactions (anaphylaxis is discussed in Chapter 6).

PATCH TESTING

Description
For this test, allergens are prepared in appropriate concentrations in white soft paraffin (e.g. Vaseline) and are then spread on to aluminium discs the size of a one pence piece. The discs (which cannot themselves provoke a reaction) are placed on your skin – usually on your back, as

shown in Figure 16 – and covered with an adhesive dressing. They are left in place for 48 hours, after which your skin is examined, and any redness and swelling are noted. Your skin will be re-examined after a further 48 hours for any remaining redness or swelling. The interpretation of this form of testing is not as simple as it sounds, and should be done only by someone with skill and experience.

Indications
Patch testing is performed in cases of contact dermatitis where allergy is suspected.

Special instructions
The symptoms of contact dermatitis must be brought under control using an appropriate steroid cream before patch testing can be carried out, or else the results will be unreliable. These steroid creams should then be discontinued for at least three to four weeks before testing, as they may suppress the test response.

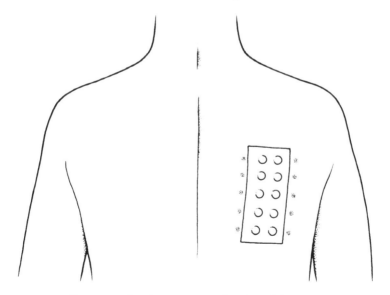

Figure 16 Patch testing on the skin of the back

Advantages
This is a relatively simple, safe and inexpensive form of testing, which is particularly useful for all forms of contact dermatitis.

Disadvantages
Interpretation of the results is not easy, and requires a thorough knowledge of your allergy history and of the materials in question. Almost 10% of the normal healthy population with no skin disease will demonstrate unexpected, apparently irrelevant, positive results. Itching or blistering may develop as a response to the test allergens.

RADIOALLERGOSORBENT TEST (RAST)

Description
This is a blood test that measures the amount of specific IgE that your immune system has produced against a particular allergen. For example, if you have asthma, it can confirm that you have antibodies against the house dust mite. (There is more information about IgE and other antibodies in the section 'Allergy explained' in Chapter 1.) Over 400 different allergens can be assessed this way.

The test is carried out on a small sample of blood taken from a vein in your arm, using a fine needle and a small syringe. Although some people dislike needles, the blood test causes minimal discomfort. The sample is then sent to a specialist laboratory, and the results are available within a few days.

RAST uses a technique in which a radioactive 'label' is allowed to attach itself to the IgE present in your blood sample. Measuring the amount of radioactivity left at the completion of the test provides information about any specific antibodies you have produced. The total amount of IgE in your blood-stream is usually measured at the same time, so that the amount of any specific IgE found can be compared to the total amount in your blood.

Indications
This test is increasing in popularity, and is often used in conjunction with skin-prick testing. It is particularly useful when the risk of an anaphylactic reaction (discussed in Chapter 6) makes skin-prick testing too risky; when extensive eczema makes skin-prick testing impractical; and when allergic symptoms are so severe that antihistamine medication cannot be discontinued to permit accurate skin-prick testing.

Special instructions
Local anaesthetic cream may be available for small children and for adults who particularly request it, to eliminate any discomfort from blood sampling. This cream takes 30 minutes to be effective, so must be applied, and covered by an airtight dressing, in advance of the test.

Advantages
This form of allergy testing is completely safe. It is specific, in that if a RAST is positive it is likely that you have a true allergy, but false negative results can occur.

Disadvantages
The test involves taking a sample of blood, which some people find unpleasant. It is expensive. A negative result does not completely rule out the possibility that allergy to the allergen exists. Do not assume that you are not at risk from a particular allergen just because the RAST is negative.

OTHER BLOOD TESTS

Multiple RAST
A form of RAST that can test for several allergens at once is now available, and is being marketed commercially through a number of large supermarkets. Because this form of testing can yield positive results when no allergy is present (false positives), as well as giving

negative results when an allergy does in fact exist (false negatives), it should not be used without the results being put in the context of a full medical history and interpreted by a doctor trained in allergy.

Other antibody tests
Although most allergy testing involves looking for evidence of the IgE antibody, in some circumstances (such as coeliac disease, discussed in Chapter 5) evidence of other antibodies such as IgA or IgG is helpful in making a diagnosis. (There is more information about these antibodies in the section 'Allergy explained' in Chapter 1.) As far as you are concerned, the test simply involves giving a blood sample as you would for RAST (as described in the previous section).

CHALLENGE TESTS

Sometimes the only way to confirm an allergy is deliberately to provoke the symptoms it causes. Challenge tests (also called provocation tests) can also be used to demonstrate that a particular allergen is not responsible for your symptoms.

Airways challenge tests

Description
You inhale increasing concentrations of either a histamine-like substance or a specific allergen solution made from the substance suspected of causing your asthma or hay fever symptoms. Your response to each dose is measured using a lung function test (described later in this appendix). The test is continued until there is a certain drop in your lung function (usually 20%). At this point, your chest may feel a little tight and you may be a little wheezy, but these symptoms will be mild. Once the test has been completed, your lung function is restored to normal by giving you a bronchodilator (reliever) inhaler to use (these inhalers are discussed in the section 'Treatment' in Chapter 2).

Indications

This form of testing is rarely used, but it can be particularly useful in the diagnosis of asthma brought on by substances encountered in the workplace. It is also used in allergy research.

Special instructions

Bronchodilator medications and drinks containing caffeine must be avoided for at least four hours before testing, and you must be free from colds.

Advantages

This form of testing can be very useful when it is helpful for your doctor to have a measurable or quantifiable response; for example, to find out if one drug suits you better than another, or to see if someone's asthma gets better when he or she stops working with a particular chemical.

Disadvantages

Although it is not painful, this procedure can be rather intimidating because of the equipment used, and requires a high degree of co-operation from the person being tested. Because of this, it cannot usually be performed on children under 7 years old. If an allergen is used, you will be kept under observation for at least eight hours after the test. There is a small risk of a severe asthma reaction, so this form of testing will be performed only by an experienced practitioner who has the facilities available to handle emergencies. These tests are relatively time-consuming and therefore expensive.

Oral challenge tests (food challenges)

Description

The food or foods suspected of causing allergic reactions are eliminated completely from your diet. If your symptoms disappear, these foods are reintroduced one at a time, at intervals of at least three days, to see if your symptoms recur. Foods are often reintroduced in capsule form so that you don't know which food is which (this is called a 'single-blind challenge'). This is to make sure that your ideas on what causes your symptoms cannot bias the results. Even better is the form of challenge in which neither you nor your doctor knows which food is being reintroduced (a 'double-blind challenge'). In a double-blind challenge, someone who is not involved with the testing process keeps the records.

Indications
This form of testing can be useful when food allergy has been previously diagnosed using inappropriate or invalid tests; when your symptoms are not typical of an allergy but may be due to food intolerance; or when several skin-prick test results are positive and it is unclear which of the foods tested is causing your symptoms.

Special instructions
This form of testing should never be performed on anyone who has suffered an anaphylactic reaction due to food allergy (anaphylaxis is discussed in Chapter 6).

Advantages
Double-blind food challenge is extremely reliable; if an allergy is present, symptoms will appear when the food responsible is introduced. If no symptoms occur, allergy can be ruled out.

Disadvantages
There is a risk of severe allergic or anaphylactic reactions, so this form of testing should be carried out only in a hospital by expert and experienced medical staff who are fully trained and equipped to handle emergencies.

LUNG FUNCTION TESTING

Two forms of lung function test are commonly used in the diagnosis of asthma, both of which simply involve you blowing out air as hard and as fast as you can into a mouthpiece connected to a piece of equipment. Full lung *spirometry* (which measures how quickly and efficiently you can empty your lungs) is generally carried out in a hospital, because the equipment required is relatively expensive, but some GP health centres now have this facility. Peak expiratory flow testing, which is described here, is more commonly used because the measuring device is not expensive and you can do it at home.

Peak expiratory flow testing

Description

This test is also known as 'peak flow testing' or 'peak flow monitoring'. It uses a peak expiratory flow meter (more usually called a peak flow meter), which is a small hand-held device that measures how fast air can be blown out from your lungs. If you have asthma, not only will your readings be lower than those of people without asthma who are of your age, height and gender (all things that affect the readings) but your readings will also be more variable from day to day. One-off readings are therefore not particularly helpful, so you will usually be given your own meter and asked to keep twice-daily recordings on a special chart, recording the best of three readings each time.

To make a reading, you take a full deep breath in, place the instrument between your lips so that an airtight seal is made between your lips and the mouthpiece, and then you blow through the device as hard and as fast as you can. Air passing through the meter moves a small pointer across a scale, indicating the maximum flow achieved. The pointer must be reset before each blow.

Indications

Peak flow recordings can be useful in the following situations:

- to aid in the diagnosis of asthma;

- to judge whether a particular treatment is or is not leading to improvement;

- to help judge the need for increased treatment if your asthma is going out of control;

- if you find it difficult to judge how bad your asthma is;

- in asthma research.

Special instructions
You should have your own device, because readings can vary slightly between meters. The device should be cleaned regularly according to the manufacturer's instructions. You should be taught how to use the meter correctly, and your technique should be reviewed regularly by your doctor or practice nurse.

Advantages
Peak flow meters are relatively inexpensive, and can be prescribed by your doctor. They can provide information that can be extremely helpful in the day-to-day management of asthma. For example, you and your doctor or asthma nurse can agree on a self-management plan (action plan), which will allow you to use your peak flow readings to judge the amount of treatment you require, and to take steps to deal with any changes in your symptoms without the need to call for medical help each time.

Disadvantages
Peak flow recordings should not be used as the sole indicator of how good or bad your lungs are on any particular day – the meters are not infallible, so you should also take note of how your chest feels and what symptoms you are experiencing. It is possible to cheat with a peak flow meter, producing both falsely high and falsely low recordings by using the wrong technique.

SYMPTOM DIARIES

Description
Your doctor or nurse may ask you to keep a record both of your symptoms and of the factors thought to be causing them; for example, a record of your bowel symptoms together with a list of all the foods you have eaten. Sometimes special forms are provided, but an ordinary notebook will do.

Indications
A symptom diary can be an invaluable source of information in almost any allergy problem.

Special instructions
Your doctor will explain to you exactly what is required, but you should feel free to include any extra information that you think might be helpful.

Advantages
People who suffer from allergy problems are often completely well on the days on which they see their doctors! It is therefore extremely useful to be able to take with you a record of how frequent and how serious your problem is, what form it takes and what might be provoking it.

Disadvantages
Not only is a symptom diary subjective, it also requires you – if it is to be of any use – to be totally honest and comprehensive when recording your exposure to allergens and any possible resulting symptoms. It may take many weeks to record enough details to provide useful information and this can require considerable effort on your part. Symptom diaries can also be difficult to interpret.

BOWEL BIOPSY

Description
In order to diagnose coeliac disease, a bowel biopsy (biopsy of the small intestine) is necessary, and there are two ways in which this can be done. The method chosen will depend on which technique is preferred at the hospital you attend. Both methods obtain a small piece of bowel lining, which can then be examined under a microscope.

The first method uses an instrument called a gastroscope, which is a flexible tube-like viewing instrument that uses fibreoptics to allow the doctor to see the inside of your digestive system. The gastroscope is inserted through your mouth into your stomach or small intestine, and the bowel lining is biopsied once the instrument is in the correct position. This technique is generally used in adults.

The second method involves a small (less than 1 cm long) capsule called a Crosby capsule, which is attached to a very fine hollow tube. Again, this is passed into the intestine via the mouth. Once it is in the correct position (confirmed by an X-ray), the capsule is triggered to take a small amount of the bowel lining, and then gently withdrawn. This technique is more commonly used in children.

Although both these procedures may seem rather unpleasant, they are not actually as bad as they sound. They are usually tolerated well, even by very small children. You will be given a sedative to help you relax while the test is being carried out.

It is essential that coeliac disease is diagnosed accurately using one of these biopsy techniques, because the treatment involves life-long avoidance of all foods containing gluten. This strict diet is not something that anyone would want to have to follow unnecessarily.

ENVIRONMENTAL TESTING

This is a test on your surroundings, not on you. A number of substances found in the environment – both at home and at work – can cause allergy problems. Occasionally it is helpful to send for analysis samples of dust, air or chemical substances used at work. This type of testing can be done only by a specialist allergy centre.

OTHER TESTS

Practitioners of complementary/alternative therapies often use diagnostic tests other than the ones I have described above. These tests are not felt by conventional medical practitioners to be relevant, standardised or repeatable, and are considered to have no place in the diagnosis of true allergy. They include the following.

- **Applied kinesiology** This measures muscle strength before and after exposure to a suspected allergen.

- **Auricular cardiac reflex method** Close proximity to a substance to which a person is allergic is said to result in a change in position in the strongest pulse at the wrist.

- **Hair analysis** The subject's hair is examined and medical problems are diagnosed from the appearance and content of the hair.

- **Leucocytotoxic tests** White blood cells are put into contact with the suspected allergen and the cells are observed under a microscope for changes in size and shape. These changes are regarded as an indication of the cells' reactivity.

- **Neutralisation–provocation testing (the Miller technique)** The dose of an allergen that can switch off or neutralise the allergy is found, and this dose is administered as drops under the subject's tongue.

- **Vega testing** This measures the electromagnetic fields produced by the subject, using a Vegatest machine.

Appendix 2 – Useful addresses

Allergy UK (formerly **British Allergy Foundation**)
3 White Oak Square
London Road
Swanley
Kent BR8 7AG
Helpline: 01322 619898
Website: www.allergyuk.org
Booklets, leaflets, quarterly newsletter, support group network. A helpline for advice and information.

Anaphylaxis Campaign
The Ridges
2 Clockhouse Road
Farnborough
Hampshire GU14 7QY
Tel: 01252 542029 (01252 318723 after office hours)
Website: www.anaphylaxis.org.uk
A charity set up to provide information, help and support for people who have life-threatening allergic reactions to peanuts and other foods.

Asthma Society of Ireland
26 Mountjoy Square
Dublin 1, Ireland
Tel: 00 353 1 878 8511
Website: www.asthmasociety.ie
Support association for people with asthma and their families in the Republic of Ireland.

Asthma UK
Summit House
70 Wilson Street
London EC2A 2DB
Adviceline: 08457 01 02 03
Supporter & Information Team: 020 7786 5000
Tel: 020 7786 4900
Website: www.asthma.org.uk
Support association for people with asthma and their families in the UK.

BBC Health
Website: www.bbc.co.uk/health
The website has an excellent section on complementary therapies.

Coeliac UK
Suites A–D
Octagon Court
High Wycombe
Buckinghamshire HP11 2HS
Helpline: 0870 444 8804
Tel: 01494 437 278
Website: www.coeliac.org.uk
Aims to improve the lives of people living with the condition through support, campaigning and research. Provides leaflets and books, and runs voluntary groups around the UK.

Education for Health
(formerly the **National Respiratory Training Centre**)
The Athenaeum
10 Church Street
Warwick CV34 4AB
Tel: 01926 493313
Website: www.educationforhealth.org.uk
Runs courses for health professionals on respiratory and allergy care and helping patients stop smoking.

National Eczema Society
Hill House
Highgate Hill
London N19 5NA
Tel: 020 7281 3553
Website: www.eczema.org
Provides practical help, information and support for people with eczema and their families.

NHS Direct
Tel: 0845 4647
Textphone: 0845 606 4647
Website: www.nhsdirect.nhs.uk
A 24-hour helpline offering confidential health-care advice, information and referral service 365 days of the year.

NHS24
Tel: 08454 24 24 24
Textphone: 18001 08454 24 24 24
Website: www.nhs24.com
Provides confidential telephone health advice and information service for people in Scotland.

COMPLEMENTARY THERAPIES

Acupuncture Association of Chartered Physiotherapists (AACP)
Southgate House
Southgate Park
Bakewell Road
Orton Southgate
Peterborough PE2 6YS
Tel: 01733 390007/390012
Website: www.aacp.uk.com
The regulatory body of physiotherapists who also practise acupuncture.

British Acupuncture Council (BAcC)
63 Jeddo Road
London W12 9HQ
Tel: 020 8735 0400
Website: www.acupuncture.org.uk
Professional body offering lists of qualified acupuncture therapists.

British Chiropractic Association
59 Castle Street
Reading
Berks RG1 7SN
Tel: 0118 950 5950
Website: www.chiropractic-uk.co.uk
Professional body promoting high standards in chiropractic in the UK.

British Complementary Medicine Association
PO Box 5122
Bournemouth BH8 0WG
Tel: 0845 345 5977
Website: www.bcma.co.uk
Ensures high-quality standards within the industry.

British Homeopathic Association
Hahnemann House
29 Park Street West
Luton LU1 3BE
Tel: 0870 444 3950
Website: www./trusthomeopathy.org
For a list of qualified homeopathy practitioners.

British Hypnotherapy Association
67 Upper Berkeley Street
London W1H 7QX
Tel: 020 7723 4443
Website: www.hypnotherapy-association.org
Maintains a list of practitioners trained to the Association's standards.

British Medical Acupuncture Society
The Administrator, BMAS
3 Winnington Court
Northwich
Cheshire CW8 1AQ
Tel: 01606 786782
Website: www.medical-acupuncture.co.uk
Provides a comprehensive list of trained acupuncture practitioners in the UK.

British Osteopathic Association
Langham House West
Mill Street
Luton LU1 2NA
Tel: 01582 488455
Website: www.osteopathy.org
Professional organisation of osteopaths in the UK; provides search facility to locate osteopaths in the UK.

British Reflexology Association
Monk's Orchard
Whitbourne
Worcester WR6 5RB
Tel: 01886 821207
Website: www.britreflex.co.uk
For a list of reflexology practitioners world-wide.

General Chiropractic Council

44 Wicklow Street
London WC1X 9HL
Tel: 020 7713 5155
Website: www.gcc-uk.org
A UK-wide statutory body with regulatory powers. Maintains a register of chiropractors who meet GCC standards of professionalism.

General Hypnotherapy Register

PO Box 204
Lymington SO41 6WP
Tel/Fax: 01590 683770
Website:
www.general-hypnotherapy-register.com
For a list of registered therapists in the UK.

General Osteopathic Council

Osteopathy House
176 Tower Bridge Road
London SE1 3LU
Tel: 020 7357 6655
Website: www.osteopathy.org.uk
Regulatory body that offers information to the public and lists of accredited osteopaths.

Institute for Complementary Medicine

PO Box 194
London SE16 1QZ
Tel: 020 7237 5165
Website: www.l-c-m.org.uk
A registered charity that provides the public with information on complementary medicine. It administers the British Register of Complementary Practitioners (BRCP).

National Council of Hypnotherapy

PO Box 421
Charwelton
Daventry NN11 1AS
Tel: 0800 952 0545
Website: www.hypnotherapists.org.uk
Maintains a register of independent hypnotherapists in the UK.

National Institute of Medical Herbalists

Elm House
54 Mary Arches Street
Exeter EX4 3BA
Tel: 01392 426022
Website: www.nimh.org.uk
Professional body representing herbal medicine practitioners; promotes the benefits of herbal medicine.

Register of Chinese Herbal Medicine
Office 5, 1 Exeter Street
Norwich NR2 4QB
Tel: 01603 623994
Website: www.rchm.co.uk
Regulatory body for the practice of Chinese herbal medicine.

Scottish Massage Therapists' Organisation
70 Lochside Road
Aberdeen AB23 8QW
Tel/Fax: 01224 822960
Website: www.scotmass.co.uk
Maintains a register of massage therapists.

Society of Homeopaths
11 Brookfield
Duncan Close
Moulton Park
Northampton NN3 6WL
Tel: 0845 450 6611
Website: www.homeopathy-soh.com
Organisation of professional homeopaths.

UK Buteyko Breathing Centre
85 Julian Road
West Bridgford
Nottingham NG2 5AL
Tel: 0115 846 1654
Website: www.buteyko.org.uk
A method to restore correct breathing.

EQUIPMENT MANUFACTURERS AND SUPPLIERS

ALK–Abelló
2 Tealgate
Hungerford
Berkshire RG17 0YT
Tel: 01488 686016
Website: www.epipen.co.uk
EpiPen suppliers.

Clement Clarke Ltd
Edinburgh Way
Harlow
Essex CM20 2TT
Tel: 01279 414969
Website: www.clement-clarke.com
Peak flow meters.

Dunlopillo Ltd
Station Road
Pannal
Harrogate
North Yorkshire HG3 1JL
Tel: 01423 877700
Website: www.dunloplatexfoam.com
Latex foam mattresses and pillows.

Medic-Aid Ltd
Heath Place
Bognor Regis
West Sussex PO22 9SL
Tel: 0870 770 3434
Website: www.medic-aid.com
Nebulisers, compressors, face-masks and spacer devices.

UCB Pharma Ltd
208 Bath Road
Slough
Berkshire SL1 3WE
Tel 01753 534655
Anapen adrenaline injectors.

Vitalograph Ltd
Maids Moreton House
Buckingham MK18 1SW
Tel: 01280 827110
Website: www.vitalograph.co.uk
Peak flow meters.

Identification jewellery

Golden Key
1 Hare Street
Sheerness
Kent ME12 1AH
Tel: 01795 663403
Identification bracelets and necklaces, for individuals with medical conditions and allergies.

MedicAlert Foundation
1 Bridge Wharf
156 Caledonian Road
London N1 9BR
Tel: 0800 581420
Website: www.medicalert.org.uk
Identification bracelets or necklaces, for individuals with medical conditions and allergies.

SOS Talisman
Talman Ltd
PO Box 985
Newton Mearns
Glasgow G77 6UY
Tel: 0141 639 7090
Website: sos-talisman.com
Bracelets, pendants, watches etc. with medical history given so that emergency services can act accordingly.

OTHER USEFUL ADDRESSES

ASH (Action on Smoking and Health)
102 Clifton Street
London EC2A 4HW
Helpline: 0800 169 0169
Tel: 020 7739 5902
Website: www.ash.org.uk
Provides information about how smoking affects medical conditions.

Department for Education and Skills (DfES)
Publications Centre
PO Box 5050
Annersley
Nottingham NG15 0DJ
Tel: 0845 602 2260
Website: www.dfes.gov.uk
For copies of DfES publications. Publications are also available online (for Managing Medicines in Schools and Early Years Settings: www.teachernet.gov.uk/wholeschool/healthandsafety/medical*).*

Department of the Environment, Food and Rural Affairs (DEFRA)
Pollen Enquiries
Pollen Research Unit
Helpline: 0800 556677 (calls are free)
Website: www.defra.gov.uk
For recorded message giving air quality information, including a forecast of pollution levels.

Department of Health
Richmond House
79 Whitehall
London SW1A 2NF
Tel: 020 7210 4850
Health literature line:
0800 555777 (calls are free)
Website: www.dh.gov.uk
Government department involved with policy making and health service issues.

Department for Work and Pensions
Olympic House
Olympic Way
Wembley
Middlesex HA9 0DL
Helpline: 0800 88 22 00
Tel: 020 8795 8400
Website: www.dwp.gov.uk
Government information service offering advice on benefits for people with disabilities and their carers.

Food Standards Agency
Aviation House
125 Kingsway
London WC2B 6NH
Helpline: 020 7276 8829
Tel: 0845 757 3012
Website: www.foodstandards.gov.uk
Sets standards in relation to food issues and ensures that these are being kept by food producers and distributors and caterers. At the same address is the Food Labelling and Standards Division, regarding all matters relating to food allergy and intolerance.

Foresight Preconception
178 Hawthorn Road
West Bognor
West Sussex PO21 2UY
Tel: 01243 868001
Website: www.foresightpreconception.org.uk
Advice and counselling on preconception care.

Health Development Authority
(formerly **Health Education Authority**)
71 High Holborn
London WC1V 6NA
Tel: 020 7067 5800
Website: www.publichealth.nice.org.uk
Deals only with research now. Publications on health matters can be ordered on 0800 555 777.

Health Education Authority
(now **Health Development Authority**)

Health and Safety Executive
Rose Court
2 Southwark Bridge
London SE1 9HS
HSE Infoline: 0845 345 0055
Tel: 020 7556 2100
Book orders: 01787 881165
Website: www.hse.gov.uk
Responsible for health and safety regulation in Great Britain.

Holiday Care Service
Tourism for All
The Hawkins Suite
Enham Place
Enham Alamein
Andover SP11 6JS
Tel: 0845 124 9971
Holiday advice for people with special needs, including information on transport, insurance, oxygen supplies, etc.

Institute of Translation and Interpreting
Fortuna House
South Fifth Street
Milton Keynes MK9 2EU
Tel: 01908 325250
An independent professional association of practising translators and interpreters in the UK.

Ministry of Agriculture, Fisheries and Food (MAFF)
(now **Department of the Environment, Food and Rural Affairs**) (**DEFRA**)

National Pollen and Aerobiology Research Unit (NPARU)
University of Worcester
Henwick Grove
Worcester WR2 6AJ
Tel: 01905 855200
Website: www.pollenuk.co.uk
Provides information about pollen counts and pollen monitoring.

Prescription Pricing Authority
Tel: 0845 850 0030
(Help with Health Costs)
Website: www.ppa.org.uk
To apply for the prepayment certificate for prescriptions.

Quit (National Society for Non-smokers)
Ground Floor
211 Old Street
London EC1V 9NR
Quitline: 020 7487 3000
Information: 020 7388 5775
Tel: 020 7251 1551
Website: www.quit.org.uk
Aims to save lives by helping smokers to stop smoking.

Quitline
Helpline: 0800 002 200
(calls are free)
The free helpline service of QUIT, it helps smokers to stop by providing advice and support.

Appendix 3 – Useful publications

At the time of writing, all the publications listed here were available.

In addition to these publications, the various allergy associations, organisations, government departments and self-help groups have excellent websites, with sections on many of the health issues related to allergy conditions. Most of this information can be downloaded. The website addresses of these organisations are given in Appendix 2.

Asthma
Asthma: answers at your fingertips, 4th edition, by Mark Levy, Trisha Weller and Sean Hilton, published by Class Publishing (2006)

Skin allergies
Eczema: what really works, by Carolyn Charman and Sandra Lawton, published by Robinson (2006)
Eczema: answers at your fingertips by Dr Tim Mitchell and Alison Hepplewhite, published by Class (2006)

Hay fever
Allergy-free Gardening: a revolutionary approach to landscape planning, by Thomas L Ogren, published by Ten Speed Press (2000)

Food allergies
Food Allergies: enjoying life with a severe food allergy, 2nd edition, by Tanya Wright published by Class (2007)
Need to Know? Food Allergies, edited by Helen Stracey, published by Collins (2007)

Anaphylaxis
Life-Threatening Allergic Reactions: understanding and coping with anaphylaxis, by Deryk Williams, Anna Williams and Laura Croker, published by Piatkus Books (1997)
Anaphylaxis: a practical guide, by Philip Jevon, published by Butterworth-Heinemann (2004)

Children
Coping with Childhood Allergies, by Jill Eckersley, published by Sheldon Press (2005)

General and miscellaneous
Managing Stress, by James Manktelow, published by Dorling Kindersley (2007)

Information available on websites
There are all the ones in Appendix 2, plus:

www.allergyinschools.org.uk
A website from the Anaphylaxis Campaign, an independent charity guided by leading UK allergists. It provides helpful information for teachers, school nurses, caterers, students and parents to help children with life-threatening allergies.

www.parentscentre.gov.uk
Information and support for parents on how to help with your child's learning, including advice on choosing a school and finding childcare.
Publications include: *Special Educational Needs (SEN): a guide to the law and your rights*

www.doh.gov.uk
The Department of Health publishes a wealth of material for health and social care professionals and other stakeholders. The fully searchable publications library contains all documents published department-wide.

Almost all the material now published by the Department of Health is available in electronic format in this section. Look in the 'Publications' and the 'Frequently asked' sections. Subjects include:

A Review of Services for Allergy: the epidemiology, demand for and provision of treatment and effectiveness of clinical interventions
This report sets out the findings of a review of allergy services, which the Government undertook to carry out in its response to a House of Commons Health Committee inquiry. It identifies actions that can be taken, both at local and at national levels, to improve services. It is accompanied by supporting information, commissioned for the review, on the epidemiology and on clinical interventions for allergies. (20 July 2006)

Publications policy and guidance section
The Patient's Charter and You: a charter for England
Department of Health publication (1 January 1996)

EHIC and health advice for travellers section
Health Advice for Travellers
This section tells you how to get medical treatment abroad, including information on the European Health Insurance card (EHIC) – the replacement for the E111 (2 February 2004)

www.dwp.gov.uk
Industrial Injuries Disablement Benefit (Disease)
For information about eligibility for state benefits in connection with conditions caused by one's occupational – e.g. asthma

Index

Vietnamese food 298
viral infections 32, 81, 90
viruses 2
visual display units (VDUs) 230
vitamins C and E 75
Vividrin 138, 142; *see also* sodium
  cromoglicate
Volumatic spacer device 53, 54, 56
vomiting 16, 156, 164, 166

walnuts 167, 170
washing and drying 142, 278–9,
  286
washing powders 91, 102; *see also*
  detergents
wasp stings *see* bee and wasp stings
weaning and food allergies 159, 160
wet wrap dressings 100
wheat 157
  allergy 104, 159, 160, 167, 168,
    294
  avoiding 297
  see also coeliac disease
wheatgerm 186, 202, 297
wheezing/wheeziness 15, 17, 32,
  35, 42–3, 104, 155, 164, 166,
  190, 192
whey 295
wine, sulphites in 36, 71, 293

wood dust 220
woollen clothing 91, 100, 102, 252
workplace (occupational) allergies
  217–18
  asthma 35, 37, 40–41, 43, 218,
    222–3
  dermatitis 113, 118, 119, 219,
    224–5, 232, 233–4
  eczema 80, 235
  and employers' responsibilities
    220, 228
  eye problems 230
  getting advice 221
  and legislation 219, 225–6
  sick building syndrome 231

X-rays 86–7
Xolair 67
xylometazoline 138
Xyzal 139; *see also* levocetirizine

yoghurt 296
Yorkshire pudding 297

zafirlukast *see* leukotriene receptor
  antagonists
zip fasteners 112, 116
Zirtek 139; *see also* cetirizine
Zovirax 111

Have you found *Allergies: Answers at your fingertips* useful and practical?
If so, you may be interested in other books from Class Publishing.

**FOOD ALLERGIES: Enjoying life
with a severe food allergy** £17.99

*Tanya Wright
with Medical Adviser, Dr Joanne Clough*

Expert Dietitian Tanya Wright combines her
professional and personal experience of severe
food allergy to give you a unique source of
practical advice. In this indispensable handbook
you will learn what it is safe for you to eat and
what you must avoid. This book shows you how,
armed with the right knowledge, you can carry
on enjoying life and food, despite your allergy.

*'Required reading for those with food
allergies.'*
DAVID READING, Director,
The Anaphylaxis Campaign

**ASTHMA
Answers at your fingertips** £17.99

*Dr Mark Levy, Trisha Weller
and Professor Sean Hilton*

Asthma – the 'at your fingertips' guide contains
over 250 real questions from people with
asthma and their families – answered by three
medical experts. This handbook contains up-to-
date, medically accurate and practical advice on
living with asthma.

'A helpful and clearly written book.'
DR MARTYN PARTRIDGE, Chief Medical
Adviser, National Asthma Campaign

**IRRITABLE BOWEL SYNDROME
Answers at your fingertips** £17.99

Dr Udi Shmueli

IBS is a trying problem that can affect
confidence and lifestyle. It is also remarkably
common. All too often, relief at doctors
finding 'nothing wrong' is tempered by
frustration at the lack of solutions available.

This practical and reassuring book looks at
the science behind the symptoms, examines
possible ways of finding relief, and gives
practical advice on taking control of your
condition rather than letting it control you.

**ACNE
Answers at your fingertips** £17.99

Dr Tim Mitchell and Alison Dudley

Acne is the most common chronic skin condition
of adolescents, affecting to some extent almost
all teenage boys and girls. It tends to begin at
puberty, and while for most people it tends to
go away by the time they reach their mid-20s,
some people may continue to have acne until
they reach their 40s or 50s.

*'By far the best book I have read on the
subject.'*
PETER LAPSLEY, Chief Executive,
Skin Care Campaign

**ECZEMA
Answers at your fingertips** £14.99

Dr Tim Mitchell and Alison Hepplewhite

With answers to hundreds of questions on every
aspect of living with eczema, this book will help
you find ways to manage your own eczema – or
that of your child – to fit in with everyday
interests and activities.

*'What a joy to have a new book which is
medically accurate, wide ranging and
practical in its approach.'*
MARGARET COX, Chief Executive,
National Eczema Society

**MIGRAINE AND OTHER HEADACHES
Answers at your fingertips** £14.99

Dr Manuela Fontebasso

Written by an experienced GP with a special
interest in headache and migraine, this book
acknowledges the uniqueness of every sufferer's
experience. Communication between patient
and professional is crucial if this complex
condition is to be addressed and the best
treatment prescribed.

Reading this book will help you understand
the nature of your headache, and will give you
the confidence to be involved in all areas of
decision making.

PRIORITY ORDER FORM

Cut out or photocopy this form and send it (post free in the UK) to:

Class Publishing   **Tel: 01256 302 699**
FREEPOST 16705   **Fax: 01256 812 558**
Macmillan Distribution
Basingstoke RG21 6ZZ

Please send me urgently   *Post included*
(tick below)   *price per copy (UK only)*

☐ **Allergies – Answers at your fingertips** (ISBN: 978 1 5959 147 5)   £20.99

☐ **Food Allergies – Enjoying life with a severe food allergy**   £20.99
   (ISBN: 978 1 5959 146 8)

☐ **Asthma – Answers at your fingertips** (ISBN: 978 1 85959 111 6)   £20.99

☐ **IBS – Answers at your fingertips** (ISBN: 978 1 85959 156 7)   £20.99

☐ **Acne – Answers at your fingertips** (ISBN: 978 1 85959 073 7)   £20.99

☐ **Eczema – Answers at your fingertips** (ISBN: 978 1 85959 125 3)   £17.99

☐ **Migraine – Answers at your fingertips** (ISBN: 978 1 85959 149 9)   £17.99

TOTAL _____

Easy ways to pay

Cheque: I enclose a cheque payable to Class Publishing for £ _____

Credit card: Please debit my ☐ Mastercard   ☐ Visa   ☐ Amex   ☐ Switch

Number _____ Expiry date _____

Name _____

My address for delivery is _____

_____

Town _____ County _____ Postcode _____

Telephone number (*in case of query*) _____

Credit card billing address if different from above _____

_____

Town _____ County _____ Postcode _____

Class Publishing's guarantee: remember that if, for any reason, you are not satisfied with these books, we will refund all your money, without any questions asked. Prices and VAT rates may be altered for reasons beyond our control.